Flying With Scissors:

A Different Perspective on Childhood Cancer

-by-

Bob Wallace

"Flying with Scissors: A Different Perspective on Childhood Cancer," by Bob Wallace. ISBN 1-58939-798-3.

Manufactured in the United States of America.

Proceeds from the sale of this book benefit Arizona Camp Sunrise. For information on obtaining additional copies, or making a charitable donation, please refer to Contacts/Credits at the end of the book, or go online to
www.flyingwithscissors.com
Thank you.

Thanks:

I would like to offer unending words of thanks to all the parents, loved ones, doctors, nurses, camp directors, and counselors that contributed to this collection. I also wish to heap praise on the American Cancer Society for all they do, including organizing and running Arizona Camp Sunrise.

Most importantly, I need to thank the remarkable kids who took time out from being kids and doing "kid-stuff" to share their stories and invaluable wisdom. I am blessed to be able to call you friends.

Disclaimer:

Although we support the author's views on children and cancer, the opinions herein relating to Jell-O, flatulence, and canned meat products are strictly his own.

Thank you.

-The Editor-

Table of Contents

Preface

The Disease(s):

Cancer. Similar to words like *taxes* and *Spam*, cancer is one of those words that can catch your attention and cause a shudder to move down your spine. However, unlike the other words, cancer carries with it a tremendous fear and directly affects the life of a patient, as well as their family and friends.

Most all of us have been touched by cancer. At very least you know of famous people who have experienced cancer. Athletes like Lance Armstrong (testicular cancer), Walter Payton (cancer of the bile duct), and Mickey Mantle (liver cancer) have faced hearing the "C" word from their doctors. Entertainment icons like Eddie Van Halen (mouth/tongue cancer), and Sharon Osbourne (colon cancer) have battled the disease. Singers Kylie Minogue, Anastacia, and Melissa Etheridge have each fought breast cancer. American political figures such as former New York City mayor Rudolph Guliani (prostate cancer), US Supreme Court Chief Justice William Rehnquist (thyroid cancer), and former First Lady Jacqueline Kennedy Onassis (lymphoma) have been affected. In some way, we have *all* been touched by cancer.

The Book:

Volumes of information have been written on the horrors of cancer. In most any bookstore you'll find an entire section dedicated to the subject. Perhaps we should warn you right off that *Flying with Scissors* is not like those others. It's different, and it's fun. No, this book doesn't deny the horrors of cancer, but it doesn't dwell on them either. Mostly, this is a book about triumph. Not just one triumph, but many, many triumphs. You'll see.

Flying with Scissors takes the personal experiences and insights of children who have battled cancer and turns them into universal truths that relate to each of us. With humor and heart, the book delivers a non-traditional look at a typically solemn topic. It's like the title says: "A Different Perspective on Childhood Cancer."

The Author:

Bob believes that life should be full of adventure. A former disc jockey, turned Registered Nurse, Bob has spent the past fifteen years working in hospitals—pediatrics, ER, ICU—and traveling throughout the world with medical and surgical teams providing care to children less privileged than our own. One of Bob's most gratifying experiences, however, has been through volunteering at Camp Sunrise.

Bob is in his tenth year as a camp counselor, and incorporates his nursing skills with his extensive knowledge of midnight raids, aerodynamic food items, and flatulence. The kids, in turn, have firmly embedded themselves as role models in his life. Continually awed by their strength, and humbled by their wisdom, Bob has set out to introduce these amazing children to the rest of us.

The Camp:

Camp Sunrise is an oncology camp put on by the American Cancer Society. The picturesque site is located near the town of Christopher Creek in the Tonto National Forrest of Arizona. For over twenty summers, kids, age eight to sixteen, who have (or have had) cancer call it home.

A camp designed specially for the brothers and sisters of cancer patients is also available. Sunrise

Sidekicks gives them a chance to develop friendships with kids living with similar circumstances, plus, share in the same camp experiences as their siblings.

And younger cancer patients, along with their siblings, can attend the Summer Fun Day Camp. Designed specifically for three to seven year olds, Day Camp provides fun and support while introducing them to the Camp Sunrise family.

You and I:

This book is our introduction to the amazing kids of Camp Sunrise. *Flying with Scissors* hails these children as the true sages and superheroes they are, plus provides the rest of us with insight and wisdom regarding how to live our lives.

And, like DC Comics used to say, "It's more fun than a barrel full of genetically-altered winged monkeys!"

Enjoy.

Dustin J. Rayhorn, MD
Pediatrics
Phoenix, AZ

"When I was a child / I spoke as a child,

I wish I could remember what I said"

-Todd Snider-

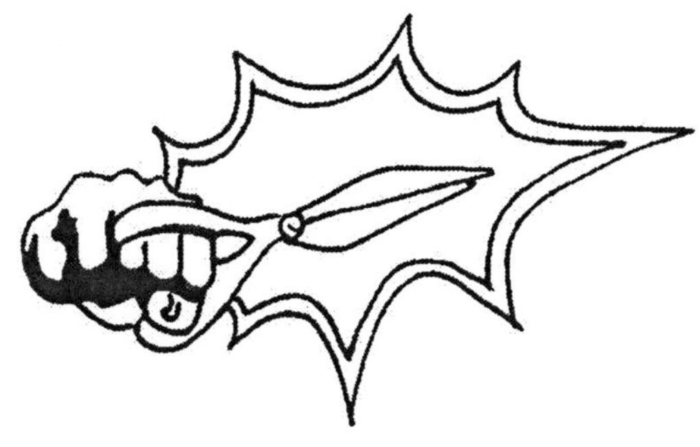

"Up, Up, and Away!"

(An Introduction:)

DC Comics introduced the world to Superman, and, soon after, gave us the Green Lantern, and the Flash. Later, Marvel Comics delivered us the Fantastic Four, the Incredible Hulk, Spider-Man, Daredevil, and the X-Men. Today, Camp Sunrise is proud to present its own syndicate of superheroes.

This alliance of modern-day superheroes is the most extraordinary association of gifted humans, rather, super-humans yet. Pitted against this new regime, the villains and evil-geniuses of the world don't stand a chance! Prepare yourselves to be amazed as we proudly present, "The Justice League of Camp Sunrise!"

But first, let's rewind nearly seventy years for a quick historical review: The Golden Age of superheroes began in 1938 with the introduction of Superman in Action Comics #1. We're all familiar with the basic storyline: Born on the doomed planet of Krypton, Superman's father shot him off in a one-baby rocket ship just seconds before the planet exploded. The rocket landed on earth (near Smallville, Illinois) where he was found and adopted by the Kents. As all good parents do, the Kents recognized the potential for both good and evil in their child's abilities, and instilled good values into their adopted son.

Clark (a.k.a. Superman) graduated high school and went to work for the Metropolis Daily Planet as a "mild-mannered" reporter. With the exception of evil-geniuses, he was well liked and dated quite a bit. (There was a mermaid named Lori and, of course, Lois Lane.) But, no matter how popular, Clark was still different. Plus, he had some intensive superhero job requirements, including the ability to change clothes quickly in a confined space, and saving the world from destruction. The job and lifestyle literally killed him (briefly in 1992), but soon he was back, and the world was again safe from evil.

Great heroes seem to attract great villains. Among others was Lex Luthor, a goal-oriented bald guy striving for both: world domination, and the demise of Superman. In addition to all the evildoers, Superman also had to deal with the radioactive chunks of kryptonite that tend to fall toward earth.

Such was his lot in life.

Superman's responsibilities made it difficult for him to lead a normal life. Although many of us have wished we were him, I'm sure there have been plenty days when Superman would rather have stayed away from phone booths, and taken the bus to his Artic Fortress of Solitude.

But this could not be—not for a superhero.

The Fantastic Four were flying an experimental rocket ship to the edge of space when the ship crashed and all four of them were bombarded by Cosmic Rays—each one forever changed by hard radiation. The mishap resulted in Reed having the ability to stretch himself to most any length, Sue could turn herself invisible, her brother, Johnny, became a human torch, and the test pilot, Ben Grimm, turned into a cynical rock-like monster-thingy.

During World War II, Princess Diana of Paradise Isle (a.k.a. Wonder Woman) showed up in her invisible jet plane wielding a golden lasso and funky-clunky golden bracelets that made her bulletproof. Wonder Woman used "force, tempered by love and justice." She was a kinder, gentler superhero. Later, she gave up her cool plane and bracelets and took up karate to keep bad guys in line.

Wimpy, lonely, and a definite geek, Peter Parker visited a science exhibit where they were giving a demonstration on radioactivity. He was unfortunate enough to be bitten by a spider that, moments prior, had been bombarded by atomic radiation. End result? Spider-strength, spider-speed, spider-agility, spider-grip, spider-sense (whatever that is), and, of course, those cool web-shooters.

It was Gamma Rays that transformed five-foot, one hundred twenty-eight pound Dr. Bruce Banner into a seven-foot tall, half-ton, green bully. A bit schizophrenic, the Incredible Hulk had super-human strength, along with some anger management issues.

The Flash had but one super-power—super-speed. Jay Garrick was never much of a football player until he broke a bunch of beakers containing gas from "hard water" and was overcome by the fumes. After that, he could walk, talk, run, and think swifter than thought itself. His newfound powers were good for chasing down crooks, as well as winning football games.

Then came a whole race of mutant children whose powers developed at puberty—the X-Men. Charles Xavier (Professor X) is the world's greatest telepath, Wolverine is a Canadian secret agent with incredible healing powers and nifty retractable metal claws, Colossus can change his body to living steel, Rogue absorbs the energy of anyone she touches, Cyclops shoots deadly power beams from his eyes, and Storm has the power to control the weather. Plus, there's a whole line of mutant villains for them to fight—the Blob, Mimic, Banshee, Saber-Tooth, Polaris, Toad—which gives the X-Men (and women) something to do when not hanging out with their friends at Mutant High.

Mathew Michael Murdock had it tough. Not only did his mom die, and a mobster kill his dad, Matt was doused by radioactive waste and rendered blind. However, the radioactivity heightened his remaining senses. He could see with a radar sense, and hear people's hearts beating to tell if they were lying. Plus, another blind guy named "Stick" taught him some slick martial arts stuff.

Mathew graduated college and started a law firm. At the same time, he adopted the identity of "Daredevil" so he could crusade against villains, in and out of the courtroom.

My favorite superhero—and possibly the one most like the kids at Camp Sunrise—is a true American icon and the scourge of the underworld: the Caped Crusader—Batman! Unlike most comic book superheroes, he is a self-made superhero. He is a spectacular crime fighter, but has no actual abilities labeled as super-human. Bruce Wayne trained his body and his mind. He is one of the few superheroes who outthinks, as well as outfights, his rivals.

To top things off, Batman has some of the funkiest gadgets around. Face it, what could be cooler than having a Bat-Plane, Bat-Copter, Bat-Mobile, Bat-Cycle, and a full crime lab all located in a huge Bat-Cave beneath your house?

That's hard to beat.

Detective Comics #190 explains "How to Be Batman." Read a little narration, study the colored draw-

ings, recite the lines from the dialog bubbles, and—
"POW! BAM! KERBOOM!" —you're a superhero!

I wish it were that easy.

What do each of these superheroes have in common? They've each suffered and conquered hardships, emerging with powers and insight well beyond normal human beings. But, as Spider-Man taught us, "With great power comes great responsibility." Some superheroes hold themselves to higher personal standards than others, but they all maintain special powers acquired from their hardships, making them unique.

Comic book superheroes have always been forced to deal with certain universal concepts such as prejudice, feeling outcast, fear of the unknown, and trying to find their place in the world. That's not unlike an adolescent, who always seems to feel somehow different. We've all wondered, "Am I the only person who feels this way?" Growing up can harbor some intense feelings of isolation.

Take a child with all the normal feelings of adolescent awkwardness and add cancer to their list of difficulties. It's mind-boggling to think that anyone could overcome such obstacles. But, in fact, thousands of kids do each year. They suffer, they conquer, and they emerge, forever changed—superheroes, each of them.

Sure, Superman can tell you what it takes to endure interplanetary space travel and the destruction of your home planet. Daredevil, the Fantastic Four, and the Hulk know what it's like to get nailed with radioactive stuff, and Spiderman will be the first to tell you that arachnoid envenomation is no fun—but did any one of them ever have to face a bone marrow biopsy?

I don't think so.

If Superman had to go through months of chemotherapy, maybe he wouldn't worry so much about kryptonite. Send a phlebotomist into Daredevil's hospital room and you'll find a fainting superhero. Even the Hulk might not think himself so incredible if he had to take medicine that he knew would leave him puking into a little plastic kidney-shaped-bowl all night long!

A comic book abbreviates into a handful of frames the trials and tribulations necessary to become a superhero. These difficulties result in the discovery of new and amazing powers. A child going through the trials of cancer, however, lives with it day-in and day-out for what can become a very long time. Often, surviving the day is their only focus, not preparing for awesome adventure.

Although not an enjoyable one, battling cancer is nothing short of an adventure. Looking back, often you can recognize a child's awesome abilities that weren't fully realized at the time. End result? Nothing less than the creation of a superhero!

All characters in this book are real; all stories true. Some of the kids have active cancer, some are in remission, some cured. Most of them are laughing, playing, acting like complete lunatics, and reveling in their childhood.

You'll find that every child sharing their story here is a not only a superhero, but an expert and a sage. The kids are here to teach us that life is made not of problems, but of dreams. And who better to show us that dreams are obtainable?

If you are a child with cancer, or were one years past, you'll no doubt have much in common with these kids. If you are a parent or loved one of a child newly diagnosed with cancer, flung headlong into an unfamiliar world, this book is a resource and companion for both you and the child you love.

Just as importantly, this book is for all of us. Children who have experienced cancer first-hand have a perspective, a certain vantage point, the rest of us rarely obtain. They can be an invaluable resource and companion to all of us.

Greetings, from **"The Justice League of Camp Sunrise!"** They have much to teach, and we, the healthy, have much to learn.

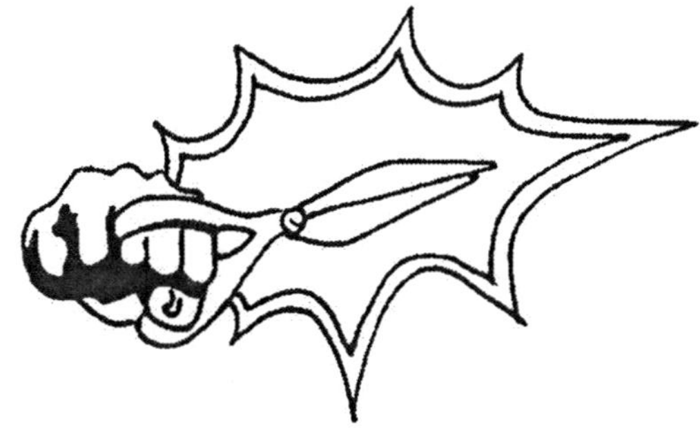

Spam

"Spam."
"Pardon me?"
"Spam."
"Spam?"
"Yes, Spam."
"Oh..."

I was submitting the topic of the class I would be teaching to our camp director, M.

"Spam?"

"Yeah...Spam."

M seemed a bit confused over my choice of classes. "So it's a cooking class?"

"Get serious," I told her, "You can't expect kids to eat that stuff—that'd be abuse."

My outline, no more formulated in my head than it was on the paper, included: Spam-Towers; Spam-Toss; Spam-Sculptures; Spam-Volcano; and my personal favorite, Aerodynamics of Spam. That one I did have figured out. I had in my possession a Spam-Launcher—a custom-made catapult device, brightly painted yellow and blue.

Having seen most everything over the years in her role as camp director, M rolled her eyes and said, "O-kay."

The first day of camp, we explain our classes to the campers, often by demonstration. The kids then choose which classes and activities they most like, and sign up for them. During this time, counselor Steve (a true Spam aficionado) and I concisely explained the many virtues of Spam.

Soon enough, the question arose, "So what's that thing?"

"This thing? This is a scientific instrument to assist in studying the aerodynamic principles of mechanically separated meat products. It's a Spam-Launcher."

"Oh," they said.

"Would you like to see how it works?"

They did.

"See those girls over there?" we asked, pointing to the yoga class diagonally across the lodge from us. "Let's pretend they are evil yoga monsters from the planet Limber."

We loaded a small cube of Spam into the palm of the backscratcher-cum-catapult lever, cleared the immediate area, and pulled the pin. The thick rubber bands went, "Thwaaap!" and the alleged pure-pork-shoulder-and-ham product launched skyward, making a beautiful arc through the heavens of the lodge. Fortunately for the unsuspecting yogis, the questionable meat product hit a crossbeam in the ceiling and fell to the floor.

Not a problem. We reloaded, recalculated the trajectory angle, and repeated the procedure. This time...success!

I wouldn't go so far as to say we were popular with the yoga-gang, but the popularity of Spam Class skyrocketed, and we had to cut enrollment off at twenty-five kids. (This was for safety reasons. When it comes to Spam, you'd hate to have things get out of hand.)

The weeklong class started out with the kids logging their guesses as to just what Spam really is. There was no winner as, to this day, we still don't know.

There was also the Spam-Easter Egg Hunt. The basic premise was to find the specially marked can of Spam hidden somewhere around camp. Return the can to Steve or myself and collect a fabulous prize, or a handful of sweet tarts, whichever we had on us. This went on all week.

Of course, we learned the "Spam Song" from Monty Python's Flying Circus. You know the one: "Spam, Spam, Spam, Spam; Spam, Spam, Spam, Spam." This, unfortunately, also went on all week long.

Thanks to the generosity of Hormel Meat Packing of Austin, Minnesota, and our friends our local Albertson's grocery store, we had ample ammunition...er, Spam—boxes and boxes of Spam. With it, we built towers. It's amazing how tall, with proper grade-school ingenuity, a tower can be engineered out of canned meat products. Later, we had the Spam-Toss. It's basically like an egg-toss, only meatier. Then came the Spam-Sculptures—amazing pieces of meat-art rivaling Michelangelo.

Next was the beautiful replica of Koo-Kuh-Tec-A-Duh-Whaka, the angry volcano. Once complete, with the assistance of vinegar and baking soda, it erupted on cue, flowing red lava down the brown meat-filled sides of the volcano.

It was fun, but didn't have the "Ohoooooooow!" factor we had hoped for. Through the kid's resourcefulness, and the use of more lava forced through a smaller hole, we were able to escalate the spew to *heights of eight feet. Now that's a volcano!*

(Author's note: If, by now, you find yourself questioning the learning aspects of Spam, I would like to point that it was taught to the kids that, like the Indians on buffalo hunts, it is important to acknowledge the sacredness of Spam. When we open a can, we use every part of the beast. To demonstrate this, the class collected all the random chunks and shavings of meat and placed them into zip-lock baggies along with notes explaining, "You've been Spammed" and "Mystery Meat for Your Feet!" These baggies somehow found their way into the foot of many a camper, counselor, and director's sleeping bag. It was a valuable lesson for the kids, and provided good feelings knowing we'd wasted nothing.)

Not meaning to gross anyone out, but, odd as it may sound, some people actually eat Spam.

I kid you not!

Take our Camp Director, M. She grew up eating Spam, and her whole family still eats it to this day. (Please don't judge them, they obviously don't know any better.) To explore this odd culinary use of Spam, we took to the kitchen. The outcome? Spam-Cupcakes with blue-tinted mashed potato frosting, of course. I can't say that anyone in the class actually tasted them, but, through the use of trickery and deceit (something the kids excel in), several unsuspecting campers got to experience the tasty cakes during snack break.

Let's not forget the Spam-Launcher. It became a daily feature of class. We would do target practice using a wastebasket at the far end of the lodge, a length of about two hundred feet. The camp sharpshooters consistently launched pink mortars that just narrowly missed the target. (What did you expect from flying meat products and a homemade catapult...a bulls-eye every time?)

We also learned much about the covert operations of Spam-Warfare. For example, pay a visit to a fresh smelling cabin (a.k.a. the Med-Shed or the Director's Cabin. Believe me, no other cabin at camp could be mistaken as "fresh smelling."). Pop a top on a can of Spam, slide it under one of the bunks, and promptly exit. Moments later, the fresh smell is magically transformed into a meaty bouquet that could be described as nothing other than "Spam-like." Mission accomplished!

Outside of learning of its many virtues at oncology camp, some of you may be wondering just what Spam and kids with cancer have in common.

My answer: Not much, and everything.

Canned meat products, like most things in life, shouldn't be taken too seriously. This, the kids taught me.

Spam makes me laugh. I mean, face it, Spam is funny! It's square—literally and figuratively. And what kind of animal is a Spam, anyway? Have you ever seen a perfectly rectangular pink critter in the wild? Not even on the Nature Channel. And, as long as we're on the topic, what is that weird slimy stuff around the meat? You know, the stuff that makes that distinctive "glug-glug" noise when you shake it out of the can?

I'm telling you, Spam is funny!

"Unless you're another Spam animal," Tim pointed out.

Good point, Tim. I stand corrected.

O-kay. So, whether you're a Spam animal, or not, it is possible you find Spam funny, unfunny, or even ugly—depending upon your point of view. That's kind of like cancer. Cancer can certainly be ugly; no one argues that. Cancer is one of the greatest struggles a person can go through—it's a life-and-death issue—and many people feel they can't, or shouldn't, even laugh around someone with the illness. But, many who have been there disagree. They'll tell you it's how you deal with a situation that can make it funny, even hilarious.

Can you imagine taking medicine that you know is going to promptly make you puke, wretch, and vomit? There's nothing funny about that, but it's the chemotherapy experience for many. Susan took that ugliness and turned it into some fun. Susan, along with her comrades-in-chemo, made it into a game. They had competitions to see who could hold out the longest before yakking.

That's ingenuity. That's turning ugly into fun. (Susan will be the first to tell you she was never very good at the game.) Taking a bad situation and finding some humor in it is a precious talent, and a beautiful art form. Given the same circumstances, I don't know that I would have the skills required.

All kids go through the self-conscious stresses of trying to fit in; it's part of growing up. Not wanting to be different is a normal concern for an adolescent. Add alopecia to that child's list of concerns, and the pressures can be staggering.

What is alopecia, you ask? It has to do with hair—namely, the lack of it. Alopecia is a fancy medical word for hair-loss, something that often comes with chemotherapy. Give a child what is ~~often~~ referred to as the "chemo cut," and it's nearly impossible for them not to stick out.

But, leave it to the kids to put things in perspective. They'll tell you that your hair falling out can be monumentally traumatic, or a great source of fun, depending upon how you look at it. Susan chose the latter response. "Losing my hair was no big deal," she says, "it was expected. And, once it's gone, you can spray paint your head—red, purple, blue—and, believe me, people look!"

Aubrie knew that her waist-length hair would soon be falling out. When that day came, she called up her friends and they came over for a head shaving party. "We had fun with it," she says. "We all took a turn in the chair, even my mother!" With a laugh Aubrie adds, "And the first swipe was always right down the middle, so there was no turning back."

"After we were all shaved, we headed down to the high school to watch the volleyball game. We really got some funny looks, fourteen bald people all walking in together."

And it didn't stop there. Aubrie's family and friends continued to shave their heads until her chemo was over and her hair started growing back. "With everyone running around bald, I knew I wasn't alone. We were all in it together," she says with a smile.

Aubrie, her mother, and her sister all took their previously waist-length hair and donated it to Locks of Love, a non-profit organization that makes wigs for cancer patients. Later, Aubrie received a wig from the same company.

Kristie remembers being 15, and in tears, as she watched her last bit of hair fall to the floor. "My friend, who routinely shaves his head, was there," she says. "He pulled out this big Hollywood-hair wig, and pointed to the two of us in the mirror, saying, 'Hey look...Sinaid O'Connor and Eddie Van Halen!'"

"Instead of crying, I found myself laughing, and we ran down the hall to show my parents. I was fine with it after that."

Kristie also donated her hair. And, as it grew back, every inch was significant. "It was like I was an inch further from where I had been with cancer." At her five-year anniversary, her hair had grown down past her waist. "I cut off two-feet and donated it again," she says, "and did it again for my ten-year anniversary."

A bit of a rebel, Kristie remembers being stuck in the hospital, awaiting diagnosis, on her 15th birthday. The doctors told her that she, either, had cancer or cat scratch disease, they weren't sure which. "I'm going down for cake," she told them, "let me know when you get it all figured out." Her obstinacy continued throughout her treatment. When her favorite oncologist would tell her to not eat pizza, she'd be sure to bring a slice to their next visit.

Missing her previously long hair, Kristie says she always wore a wig at school and many people never knew she was ill. That is, until cheerleading tryouts. Determined not to let it get her down, Kristie went from a radiation appointment straight to tryouts. "When I dumped my wig for my gymnastics routine, a lot of people thought my hair just fell off," she laughs, "but I'd taken it off myself."

Always managing to find good in a difficult situation, Kristie remembers, "I was the only freshman to get out of school early. It was pretty cool. Of course, I had to spend the time getting radiation…but still, I got out early!" Kristie missed over three hundred days of high school, but still managed to graduate on time, with a high GPA, and scholarships.

Susan, Aubrie, and Kristie are not the only ones with the ability to find fun within adversity. Far from it. Many cancer survivors echo this amazing capacity. Whether it's Nathan racing down the hospital corridor riding on his I.V. pole, or Harvey laughing while he pulls out handfuls of hair and tosses them out the car window on the ride home from chemo, the desire to enjoy life, despite the obstacles, is constant.

Laughter heals, and having fun is good for you. We all know that. (Although some of us seem to forget it as we mature.) But now scientists have joined in the fun, too. Multiple studies have shown us that a positive attitude, laughter, and fun are not just emotionally, but physically, good for you.

To many, that's like spending a few million dollars on a study that tells us, "We've found that there is a correlation between beans and flatulence."

To quote most anyone from the senior girls cabin, "Duh."

Lee Berk, Doctor of Public Health, is a professor and medical research scientist in the School of Medicine and Public Health at Loma Linda University. He is a psycho-neuroimmunologist. (Try saying that three times fast with your mouth stuffed full of marshmallows!) Dr. Berk is a pioneer and leader in conducting scientific research on mirthful laughter.[1]

In the 1980s there was already volumes of research confirming that physical and psychological stress produce chemical and neurological changes in people. However, most of the research focused on negative stress, or distress. Dr. Berk decided to study the impact of eustress, or positive emotional states. He and his colleagues looked at the biochemical changes that occur relative to the eustress state of mirthful laughter.

The research was scrupulously controlled as test subjects watched videotapes of stand-up comedians, and the control group watched travel films. Blood samples were checked before, during, and after the viewing, plus the next day.

The results were undeniable.

During mirthful laughter, there is a chemical stimulus that activates T-cells (T lymphocytes), which help the body prepare to combat viruses, bacteria, and other foreign bodies. There was also an increase in the numbers

---

[1] Patty Wooten, *Psychoneuroimmunology of Laughter: An Interview with Lee Berk, Dr. PH*, JOURNAL OF NURSING JOCULARITY, Fall 1997, 46-47 *available at* <u>www.jesthealth.com/art26jnj9.html</u>.

and activity of Natural Killer Cells (NK cells), which are a type of immune cell that attacks virally infected cells and some types of cancer and tumor cells.

They also saw increases in the antibody Immunoglobulin A (IgA), which helps fight upper respiratory problems, and an increase in the immunoglobulins IgM, IgG, and B Lymphocytes also occurred. These and other physical findings showed that mirthful laughter gives a significant boost to the immune system.

Dr. Berk says it is objective scientific data that supports the verse from Proverbs, stating, "A merry heart does good like a medicine."

As well as boosting our immune function, other studies have confirmed that humor and laughter also activate the release of endorphins, which are the body's natural painkillers. The results are plentiful, showing that fun and laughter is not just emotionally, but physically good for us.

Dr. Bob Krauth says working with children, and with the families of children, with serious diagnoses has been very rewarding to him. But his credentials go much further than that. He's a camp physician, a veteran camp counselor, and a legend when it comes to telling campfire stories. (Ask him about Rupert, but be sure you have some time on your hands.)

Discussing the amazing examples of positive attitude demonstrated by kids at Camp Sunrise, he says, "I don't know that you can develop this type of attitude toward life without going through something huge, like cancer." Dr Krauth credits the kids for his choice of career. "Without camp" he says, "I don't think I'd be a doctor today."

Lacey and Brittnee, the self-proclaimed "Fashion Queens" of the Ladybug cabin, have undeniably positive attitudes. Talk to them, even for a minute, and their infectious laughter will dissolve any concerns you may have had about your own day.

Brittnee, a beautiful eleven-year-old with corn-rowed hair, remembers her days in the hospital. "The big castle—that's what I call it—it's o-kay, but kind of scary. The nurses are pretty cool, though. Best thing of all is you can ring your call-bell anytime and they'll bring you Fruit Loops!"

Lacey, a ten-and-one-half year old high-volume, high-intensity, vibrant, redhead announces that she is celebrating her fifth anniversary of being out of treatment. "Five years, twelve hours, and some minutes," she clarifies.

To Lacey, the worst thing about being in the hospital was missing being home with her friends and family. "Ever since my treatment, I can't do contact sports, but" she adds, "I can dance and sing!"

The two of them demonstrate their skills with an impromptu concert, complete with choreography.

"Laughter helped me get through my cancer," Jason tells us. He was almost seventeen when he went through chemotherapy, surgery, then more chemo, and radiation. Jason lost all his body hair, even his eyebrows. He laughs as he remembers, "I didn't have any zits though, that was cool." He explains that chemo drugs kill everything, including acne. "That's one of the few upsides to chemo—no zits!"

Jason had most of his gluteal muscle removed from his right side, and jokes that he's done everything *half-assed* ever since. He was hairless when he finished up his Eagle Scout Merit Badge and claims to have been the only Bald Eagle in the state.

Staging an annual Jell-O War is an Camp Sunrise original, but the idea could have come from any child enduring an extended hospital stay. While inpatients at Phoenix Children's Hospital, Liz and her friend Jake kept the nursing staff on their toes. "We were the night owls," she says. The two of them acquired some fake teeth and wandered into other units posing as hillbilly hicks. "We also had silly string, whoopee cushions, and a remote control rat with red blinking eyes. The night shift nurses would be afraid to even come in our rooms!"

"Messing with the nurses helps you stay sane. Once, when feeling mischievous," she says, "I poured apple juice into the sterile specimen cup that was supposed to be for my urine sample. Just as I was handing it to the nurse, I pulled it back, looked at it closely, and said, 'It's a bit cloudy.' Then, to the nurse's horror, I drank it down!" Liz laughs and adds, "I told her it needed to be filtered one more time."

It's not just laughter that helps motivate us to heal, it's any expression joy. You don't have to go around singing the "Spam Song" to have a positive outlook, and a constant diet of full-goose belly laughs is not required to be healthy. Anything that brings you joy or makes you smile will be beneficial, both physically and emotionally.

If you learn anything from a child who's been through cancer, it's probably that, even during the worst of times, life can be a comedy, and every day provides reason to celebrate. The first Sunday in June is celebrated as National Cancer Survivor's Day, but if you were to ask the over ten million cancer survivors in this country, I think you'd find that most celebrate every day.

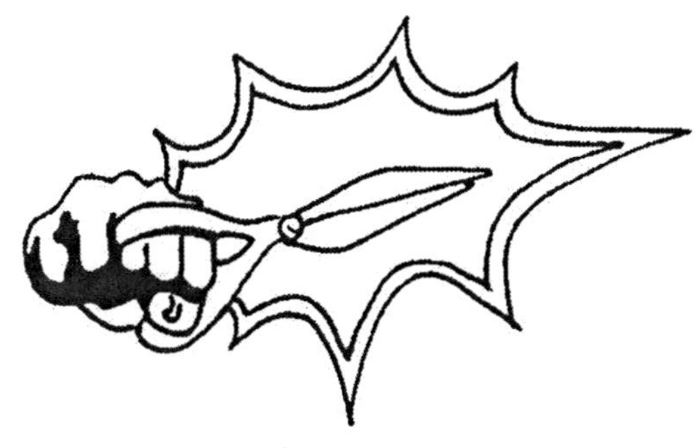

Pirates!

The picnic table in front of me magically transforms into a Spanish galleon, and the Summer Day Campers running toward it, pirates! There's no doubt about it, this rag-tag mob of three-to-seven year old swashbucklers is a force to be reckoned with. (The exception being Tracy, who is exercising her option of being a princess, complete with tiara.)

"ARRRRRRRRRRR!!!" the pirates yell.

"ARRRRRRRRRRR!" I yell.

Soon the ship is ours, and I lay down on the bench to catch my breath, knowing the next adventure will not be far off.

In the calm after the melee, I ponder. These kids—most of whom I can barely keep up with—have cancer. Every last one of them! Everyone knows that cancer is bad, but how much do most of us really understand about the disease? Maybe an overview would be appropriate—kind of a "Cancer-101" if you will.

Cancer is a whole group of diseases, which can be confusing, but they all have this in common: they all involve cells growing out of control. Renegade cells that have the ability to invade a person's body, grow, take on abnormal sizes and shapes, ignore their normal boundaries, and destroy their neighboring cells.

Our entire bodies are made up of cells—over 10 trillion cells—and, ultimately, cancer can spread (or metastasize) to other organs and tissues. Even though there are many differences in the types of cancer common to children and adults, and in the ways they are treated, all cancers fit into this same broad definition.

Muscle, bone, blood, and bone marrow (where blood is made) are all composed of cells. Cells originate from young cells that receive specific chemical messages instructing them to grow faster or slower, depending upon the body's needs. The cells reproduce, mature, and die—this is normal for cells. Once cells die they are replaced by new cells in a process called renewal.

Most cancers come from one or more young cells that have somehow lost their built-in ability to respond to the normal chemical messages telling them to mature and die. Instead, they reproduce repeatedly, replicating the same abnormalities. These cells seem to have an unlimited ability to reproduce. They are out of control. Cancer cells often reproduce so fast that they need to spread into new areas. They invade other tissues, bone marrow, or blood, and sometimes grow into tumors, which are clusters of the abnormal cells.

You might wonder, *"Is cancer common in children?"*

The answer would be no. Cancer in children is considered quite rare, actually. The chances of a child getting cancer can be
compared to that of winning the lottery—not very likely. For instance, the odds of a child developing a

neuroblastoma—a solid tumor cancer of the sympathetic nervous system—is less than one in 100,000.[2]

Let's look at it this way. If you were to attend an Arizona Cardinal football game at Sun Devil Stadium...no wait, let's make it a Diamondback baseball game at Bank One Ballpark (after all, we *do* want the seats full of fans), and everyone there was under the age of eighteen, the theoretical number of kids in attendance with a neuroblastoma would be one-half of one.

One-half—not even one child!

To theoretically have one sick child at the ballgame, we'd have to squeeze two children into every seat.

The chances of a child getting Rhabdomyosarcoma — a form of cancer affecting the soft tissue—is less than 200,000-to-one.[3] Not too likely at all. Back to Bank One Ballpark, but this time we have to fit four kids into each of the seats for the statistical likelihood of one child in attendance having the disease.

All those fans and only one kid with cancer. Not bad, eh? Statistically speaking, I mean.

"So," you may ask, *"then what's the big fuss about kids with cancer?"*

Let's ask Sabrina. She was born two months premature and only weighed three pounds. At just six months of age, Sabrina was diagnosed with a Neuroblastoma. Her tiny body housed a tumor that weighed all of two pounds. You could say that not

---

[2] Marc T. Goodman et al., *Sympathetic Nervous System Tumors, in* NATIONAL CANCER INSTITUTE: SEER PEDIATRIC MONOGRAPH 65, 71 (1999) *available at* http://seer.cancer.gov/publications/childhood.

[3] James G. Gurney et al., *Soft Tissue Sarcomas, in* NATIONAL CANCER INSTITUTE: SEER PEDIATRIC MONOGRAPH 111, 111 (1999) *available at* http://seer.cancer.gov/publications/childhood.

only did she not pick the lucky lottery ticket, she was dealt the cancer card. That made for quite a fuss.

Or, we can ask Natalie. At nine and one-half, she was an active little gymnast. Then, one day, Natalie was told she had Rhabdomyosarcoma, and that she would have to undergo surgery, chemotherapy, and radiation. To Natalie and her family, this was a big fuss.

Though the chances of these girls getting cancer were statistically quite low, they got it anyway. Isn't it just like a child to ignore the odds?

The low odds of a child contracting cancer are encouraging. In addition, children have always been more resilient and have higher cure rates than adults with the same disease. Plus, over the past twenty-five years, incredible progress has been made in the treatment of childhood cancers. The statistics are optimistic.

Medical experts tell us the mortality rates for children with cancer have decreased dramatically. Mortality has decreased for every cancer site; most by at least 50 percent.[4] Medical and statistical jargon aside, that means almost twice as many children survive cancer today.

That's impressive!

Survival rates vary, depending on the type of cancer and what part of the body it affects, but more children than ever are surviving childhood cancer. Over the past thirty years, survival into adulthood increased from thirty to eighty percent.[5]

---

[4] National Cancer Institute, *Cancer Rates Among Children Under Age 15, in* NATIONAL CANCER INSTITUTE: SEER PEDIATRIC MONOGRAPH (1999) *available at* http://seer.cancer.gov/publications/raterisk/rates31.html.

[5] NATIONAL CANCER INSTITUTE, YOUNG PEOPLE WITH CANCER: A HANDBOOK FOR PARENTS, *at* http://www.cancer.gov/cancertopics/youngpeople, accessed Jan. 16, 2005.

Leukemia accounts for almost one-third of all cases of cancer in children from birth to fourteen years of age. In the early nineteen-sixties the survival rate for children with acute lymphocytic leukemia, the most common type of childhood leukemia, was between zero and five percent.[6] The likelihood of survival increased to about 53% in the mid-seventies, and was up to 80% by the mid-nineties.[7] Today, the survival rate is expected to be even higher yet.

Some other common forms of childhood cancer sport even higher cure rates. Wilms tumor—involving the kidneys—has a 90% survival rate, and Hodgkin's Disease—a cancer of the blood—94%.

You may find yourself wondering, *"With only a fraction of children getting cancer, and with the statistics of being cured so encouraging...again, what's the big fuss about kids with cancer?"*

The fact of the matter is this: If it's your child that is the ill one, the numbers are pointless and, yes, it's a very big fuss.

Most anyone who has dealt with a child going through cancer will tell you that, when it's your own child, the statistics are either 100%, or 0%. They either make it, or they don't. Yoda summed it up. In *The Empire Strikes Back*, he said, "Try? There is no try. There is only do, or not do."

I know, I know, *"So where did all the good news and fun go?"*

That's a good question, and it's coming...

You see, having cancer can be a horrible experience for a child and those who love them, but, as we've seen, more and more children survive the experience and go on to live incredible lives. I hate to

---

[6] Malcolm A. Smith et al., *Leukemia, in* NATIONAL CANCER INSTITUTE: SEER PEDIATRIC MONOGRAPH 17, 32 (1999) *available at* http://seer.cancer.gov/publications/childhood.

[7] *Id.* at 17.

ruin the plot, or blow the punch line for you, but here's a hint—

Remember Sabrina, the one child in 100,000; and Natalie, the one child in 200,000? They were both that one ill child out of the hoards of healthy fans squeezed into the stadium seats—the ones that got dealt the unfortunate card.

The good news is that their illnesses happened a long time ago—years and years ago. It's now eighteen years later, and Sabrina is a beautiful young woman who has graduated high school. And it's been nearly thirteen years for Natalie. She has graduated college and has her sights set on law school. Both are vibrant young adults out to make a difference in the world.

Sabrina and Natalie were kids that, though the odds were against it, got cancer. And they are now young adults who beat the disease and are living lives that are active and fulfilling.

Best of all, they're not alone. Far from it!

There are thousands—tens of thousands—of kids who have done the same. Each has a unique story to tell, but all share a common bond—they are cancer survivors! It's a pretty impressive addition to life's résumé.

"Land ho!"

You'll have to excuse the interruption as my thoughts are tragically fractured, and my rest period has sadly ended.

Again, a shout comes from the crow's nest. "Button your hatches and buckle your swashes, land lubbers, we're goin' ashore!"

I'm not sure just what that means, but my fellow pirates and I are off to invade an unsuspecting plot of grass, which, before my eyes, magi-

cally transforms into a deserted island somewhere in the Caribbean.
Such is the life of a pirate.

Later, pillaging and plundering behind us, I again pause to contemplate things. I can't help but wonder, *"Why is it that, through a child's eyes, it's a world of possibilities, while for so many of us it's a world of limitations? What is it between childhood and adulthood that changes our views so drastically?"*

I'm not sure.

Possibly it has to do with belief—belief in one's self, one's abilities, and in the goodness of life.

Maybe that's one reason children do so much better in overcoming life-threatening illnesses like cancer. Possibly their belief and expectations of overcoming the illness and getting on with the good things in life are a prime factor in their success. Likewise, possibly the disbelief and negative expectations of many adults is a key factor in their less favorable results.

When posed with the choice of setting your dreams and imagination flying, or tying them to an anvil and throwing them in the fishpond, kids are likely to choose the first option. Adults, on the other hand...well, the choice is up to us.

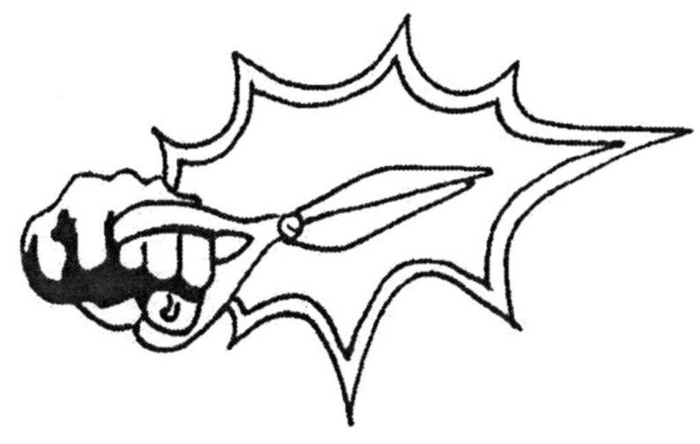

Cancer Envy

After successfully trading away several lunch items, as well as my lanyard and a monkey fist, I've successfully amassed a collection of no less than seven chocolate chip cookies.
Not a bad day's work.
The cookies sit stacked in a precarious tower of baked goodness. Yes, the barter system is alive and well at Camp Sunrise!
I'm beaming over my treasure, feeling good about myself, as Kelsey—one of the children I relieved of their cookies—asks, "Uncle Bob, what kind of cancer did you have?"

I sit quietly, searching for an adequate answer. My palms dampen and a rush of shame drains all pigment from my face. What kind of cancer did I have? Busted! Time to fess up—game over.

"Uh...I'm sorry Kelsey, but I...I didn't actually have cancer..." I feel exposed and wholly inadequate—my secret revealed, "...of any kind," I add.

"Oh," she replied nonchalantly, "I thought we all did."

Unaffected, Kelsey retuned to munching on a French fry, one she liberated from my tray during our bartering.

What? Did I really say that? *"I'm sorry, but I don't have cancer!"* No way, that's ridiculous.

I did say it.

Although I would never actually wish to have cancer, or any other disease, more than once I've found myself besot with "cancer envy." It's kind of a peer pressure reversal. It sounds odd, for certain, but it's as real as they come.

When in the presence of a true superhero, such as Kelsey, it can leave you feeling small—very small. These are children who looked terror in the eye and walked on past. They are young adults who battled for their life and won. These are superheroes, every one.

Kelsey is only 10, and small for her age. She's a little angel sitting on a bench eating french fries from her lunch tray. She's unassuming—yes. But trifling? juvenile? immature?—not even close.

Kelsey is a veteran of life and has experienced so much that I, thankfully, have not. At her young age, Kelsey has battled and ultimately conquered death, only to sit seemingly unscathed nibbling a french fry. Like mild mannered Clark Kent, before going into a phone booth, she's the epitome of modesty.

I looked around the lunchroom and saw similar faces everywhere. Each unique, yet each housing some discrete authority missing in my own. I saw an entire lunchroom of them, some barely surpassing my beltline, but all united in their entitlement of being dubbed "Superheroes."

Feeling insignificant, I passed my entire tower of cookies onto Kelsey's tray and told her, "Here, these are for you. You earned them."

As for me, I have a lot yet to accomplish before I could ever be so entitled.

Walking away, I noticed Kelsey smiling and passing out cookies to a whole table full of pint-sized superheroes.

As it should be.

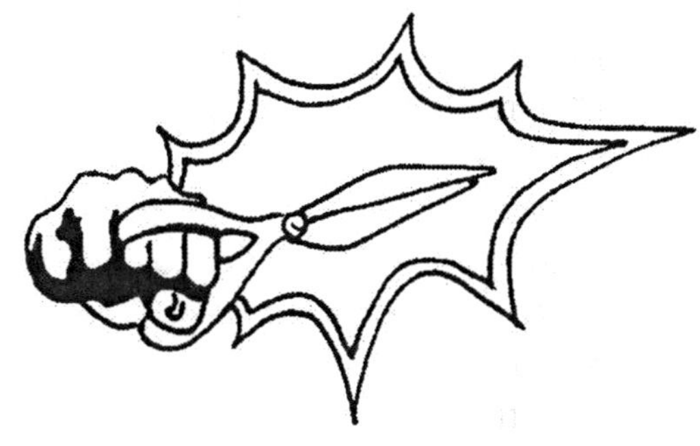

Warfare

It's dark—really dark. The silent forest envelops me and hides me from sight. At least, I hope it does. The darkness is thick, dense, almost overwhelming. A couple flashlights wink in the distance, then disappear. My own breathing is the only thing audible, backed by the internal thump of my racing heartbeat—lub-dub, lub-dub, lub-dub—like a giant sub-woofer in one of those cars that go "boom."

I've got to find Ralphie. Find Ralphie. I creep slowly forward on all fours. A twig snaps to my left, and I fall to my belly—silent. That eerie feeling that I'm being watched wriggles its way into the back of my mind. I try to dismiss it.

Find Ralphie.

Crawling forward on my stomach, I feel every rock and twig. Where's Ralphie? I'm unprotected behind enemy lines with not even a water pistol.

It's slow moving but I can see the enemy encampment. Two, three...it looks like four of them sitting on the flag. This game will never end! Hanging off belt loops, two of the guards have glow-sticks giving off eerie green illumination. "Not too stealthy," I think, "amateurs." I can make out Kyle in the distance. He's small, agile, and extremely fast—a dangerous combination. Just beyond the glow-sticks, I hear Steve's voice from atop the picnic table, which serves as the jail.

"Hello, Dad—I'm in jail!" He's chattering lyrics from a Was Not Was song, encouraging us to come to his rescue, plus, it doubles as a distraction, buffering any noise we may make while trying to get close. What a pro.

"Happy Birthday Dad, I'm in jail!"

One jailer sports a pair of night-vision goggles, as he has, day-and-night, all week. I find myself pondering, "Do those things really work?" And then, "I wonder where I can get a pair?"

Suddenly, a shadow bolts from the darkness to my right.

It's Ralphie, he's going for it! Suicide!

Running interference, Ralphie sprints out in the open, luring three of our opponents away from the flag. It's time to make my move.

As I rise to a crouch, I hear Steve yell, "Run, Ralphie, run!" all the while he's waving me to go for the flag. The guard has his back to me, the flag is exposed, and I sprint with all I've got.

"I'm fast. I'm fast," I think, "Nothing but stealth."

Blosh!!! I take one from behind, and feel the cold water ooze down my back. But still, I run.

"Focus, focus on the flag—you're almost there."

Without warning, a small hand grasps my forearm, "Gotcha, Uncle Bob!"

Darn. Run down by a nine-year-old—again!

As I am led to the picnic table/jail, out of breath, I'm afraid I might vomit. No, not from the water balloon I took in the back, but from the burrito bar at dinner. I shouldn't have taken thirds.

Ralphie is waiting for me at the picnic table, already incarcerated. "War is heck, Uncle Bob," he says, and shoots me with my own squirt gun.

"Ughh," is all I can muster in response.

So often terms of warfare are associated with illness. Fighting a bug... Battling a cold... Combating the flu... The war against cancer!

There it is, cancer.

The big "**C**."

The fight against cancer has gone on for a long time. The medical field began studying cancer at least as far back as the 1600s, and has been engaged in a full-scale battle for many years now.

Some feel that, within a few years, cancer treatment will be so radically advanced that our current forms of treatment will be looked on with the same disdain we allot the bloodletting of medieval times.

Let's hope so.

Currently, doctors head a multi-faceted team of professionals—surgeons, oncologists, nurses, scientists, laboratory personnel, child-life specialists, and social workers—as they hunt down the cancerous enemies, wherever they may lurk. They infiltrate the foreign troops and use whatever measures necessary to eradicate them.

Often, weapons of mass destruction, the really "Big Guns," are used to wreak havoc on the cancer, but, at the same time, they can adversely affect multiple organs and systems in the body. These weapons, and their after-effects, can alter a person physically, mentally, and emotionally.

After the battle, we use close surveillance to watch for any factions of the invading cancer attempting to reform. If necessary, we launch another attack. At the same time, we do everything possible to support and recuperate our bodies, rebuilding them to be the healthy unit they were prior to the invasion.

Just like any war, casualties can be high. Unfortunately, the "weapons of mass destruction"—chemotherapy, radiation, etc.—obliterate healthy cells as well as cancerous cells without discrimination. Collateral damage can be extreme.

Anyone who has been involved in the battle can attest to the truth of Ralphie's statement, "War is heck." Aggressive destruction and violent annihilation does not paint a very pretty picture, but war rarely is pretty. For cancer patients, that is the battle at hand.

For now, anyway.

The good news is that, although tolls have been high, we are gaining ground each year. Cancer treatments have progressed, drugs to minimalize negative side effects have seen huge advancements, and outcomes have improved drastically.

In the future, we trust that all children will be afforded a life of peace and harmony, free from disease. But, for now, the war continues.

It's no game, but fortunately, many thousands of children are winning the battle. Each year, more and more are claiming victory, putting it behind them, and living lives that are long, productive, and fulfilling.

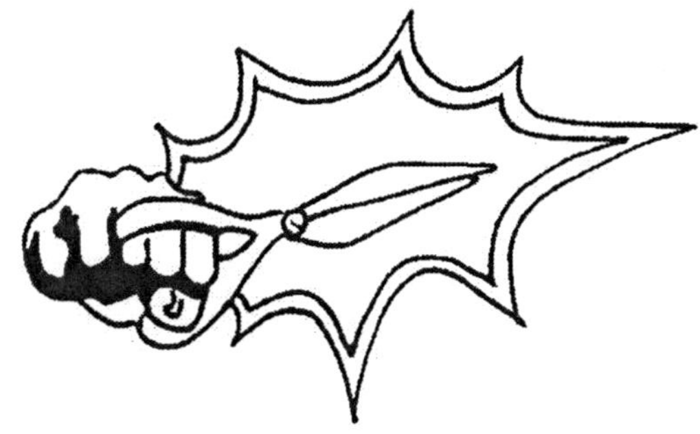

You are Not Your Disease

Down at the swimming hole, the kids are rhyming off their cancers as if they were right out of a Dr. Seuss book:
    "Non-Hodgkin's Lymphoma..."
    "Neuroblastoma..."
    "Rhabdomyosarcoma..."
    "Pharyngioma..."
    "Manangioma..."
    "Astrocytoma..."
    "Retinalblastoma..."
    "Osteosarcoma..."

How is it that these young children have a medical vocabulary rivaling a seasoned MD? Why is it that, so early in life, their maturity made such a quantum leap?

Cancer...oh yeah, cancer. These kids have been through cancer!

It's true. You walk around camp with hordes of over-stimulated kids—running, screaming, and acting a fool—and you forget the very thing that brought them all together. They've all had cancer. You'd never know it from most of them, until they get to the swimming hole, strip down to their swimsuits, and start comparing scars.

"That's where my spleen burst."

"I've had so many spinal taps that my mom jokes that you can play connect-the-dot on my back."

"Spinal taps? How many bone marrows have you had?"

"That's nothin', they cut me wide open... twice!"

"These kids can tell you what white counts mean. And about neutrophils, lymphocytes, and platelets. Plus, how they all affect each other." Dr Bob Krauth smiles, "Things I have difficulty explaining."

Natalie remembers flushing her own central line catheter and changing her own dressings. She always knew what her platelet, hemoglobin and hematacrit counts were, and when she was in need of a transfusion. She also knew her chemotherapy drugs and their side effects, and she wasn't afraid to ask questions of the doctors.

"I'd get all upset when the doctors and my parents would be in the room whispering. I'd cut in and say, 'O-kay, I know you're talking about me. So either come over here and talk, or step out of my room!'"

She continues, "There's a Yiddish phrase, 'Children have big ears.' Kids know what's going on, so just be up front with them, because they usually know it anyway."

When a doctor first utters the diagnosis of cancer, parents are often unable to comprehend it. How could such a horrid disease attack their precious child? At times, the child deals with it much better than the parent.

At four months age, Noah was diagnosed with retinoblastoma, a tumor of the eye. His mother remembers receiving the news, "When a doctor tells you your child has cancer, you hear everything they say, but you don't necessarily register it; you're kind of in a zone. The doctor said, 'it needs to come out,' and I thought, oh God, surgery on the eye, that's serious. Then he said, 'No, the *eye* has to come out.'" "I was crushed. His cancer took over," she says, "it became my life."

After six surgeries over a two-year-and-four-month time period, Noah is doing well. He has a prosthetic eye that looks natural, and he is as active as any three year old. His mother, meanwhile, has gone on to help many other parents in similar situations.

Liz was fifteen and far from ready to let any illness slow her down. She needed to be admitted to the hospital, but refused until after the final matinee of her junior high play.

Following the final bow, they rushed her to the hospital for a needle biopsy and ended up draining two liters of fluid from her lungs. By that evening, she had a chest tube and was diagnosed with Non-Hodgkin's Lymphoma.

"At fifteen I didn't even know what cancer was, or that anyone but old people got it," she says. "I was getting into teenagerdom, and was probably a little arrogant, but you can't take it all on your own, you need support. Even if you think you're the toughest person, like I thought I was, you're going to need others."

As for the battle wounds a person endures, Liz quotes a hospital friend and fellow cancer survivor: "Scars are like tattoos, only with better stories."

Bobby's mom relates, "It's heart-wrenching to look back at where we've been, but now we're looking forward to his teenage years."

She says it can be hard to disengage from the overprotective mindset. "It's kind of tough on me," she says. "We did everything together while we were going through his treatments, so we have a real special bond. He's pretty much healthy now, and independent, and doing his own thing, and has that teenage attitude, you know?" With a laugh she admits,

"It's hard on me, but it's a natural detachment, which is healthy, and I try not to hover over him."

Seeing Bobby today, with his curly brown locks, it's hard to imagine him hairless, as he was when he first came to camp. His smile being his one consistent feature.

As an infant Sabrina went through four different surgeries, and in every one of her baby photos she has tubes connected to her. She says that, even in photos from when she was four or five, her hair still hadn't all come in. At the time, it made her insecure around other kids. Nowadays, she's anything but shy, and says she still feels overprotected. "The only girl in the family *and* I had cancer...I'm waaaay over-protected!"

Kelsey was 2½ when she was diagnosed with a neuroblastoma—not an easily curable form of cancer. Kelsey's mom says that the first two weeks after her daughter's diagnosis, she lived in a total haze. Then she decided she was going to dive in, learn everything she could, and be an advocate for her child. "You need to educate yourself and just go for it," she says.

"This is the worst thing you could ever face as a parent and it's easy to get paralyzed with your own fear," she warns. "Don't disengage; don't hide from it and hope it will go away. Jump in with both feet, learn everything you can, and stay positive, because that outlook is healthy for your child."

For ten months Kelsey endured chemotherapy, radiation, and a bone marrow transplant. Later, with the news that the cancer had returned, things looked bleak.

Kelsey was referred to a specialist in Denver and underwent surgery. Things appeared to be going well, but the cancer again returned. Doctors told the family that there was nothing else that could be done. Kelsey, their precious child, was given less than six months to live.

Refusing to accept this prognosis, her parents did not give up hope. "You must stay positive no matter what," her mom says, "I believe that, and I believe in prayers."

Traveling to Sloan Medical Center in New York City, Kelsey was accepted into a Phase-II Clinical Trial involving Monoclonal Antibodies. "It worked!" Mom reports proudly, "She's been cancer-free for almost five years now."

"We never gave up. If we had taken the word in 1999 that she only had six months to live...I don't know where we would be today."

She is quick to admit that overprotecting your child can be a natural reaction. "They told me I couldn't keep her in a bubble, and I thought they were nuts. But my husband and I talked, and realized that you can't give up quality for quantity."

Steve agrees, "You wanna live life. You realize that something bad could happen, and you want to use caution, but you don't want to worry every second for the rest of your life. You got to live it up, because you only get one!"

Getting past fear is one of the largest challenges for the parent of a child with cancer. "I had a great independent early childhood," Natalie explains, "Then, when I got cancer, my mom went from being a pretty laid-back parent to an overbearing, overprotective, overly cautious mom. She'd tell me 'No, no, no, no' to everything. She was just scared. I do think that sometimes, to this day, she still sees me as a nine-year-old in need of help."

"It's really not fair," Dr. Krauth explains, "that a six-year-old can have been through so much that now he acts more like an adult than many adults do. The people who run the treatment centers work hard to allow kids to stay kids...just like at camp."

At first, Susan was given only a ten percent chance of living. "I told my parents not to cry. And I asked all the hard questions at first—'Am I going to live? Am I going to be paralyzed for life?'—my parents were just too upset."

Susan is doing fine now, and says, "It's good to have my parents treating me regular again."

A family role-reversal is not uncommon. "In the time it takes to have an MRI," Jeremy tells us, "I went from a healthy active life to, 'Bam!,' I have a brain tumor. Next thing I knew, instead of driving my younger brother to baseball practice, he was transporting me to treatments."

Michelle is a veteran camp counselor who is currently in graduate school for clinical psychology. It is her life's desire to help children cope with cancer. "Not just the ill child," she says, "but the parents and siblings too. Parents feel helpless, and, at times, it's instant maturation for the child. Plus, the brothers and sisters of a cancer patient can feel totally left out, and have their own particular needs."

With all the attention going toward the child with cancer, it's not surprising that siblings can feel lost in the shuffle. Understanding this, the American Cancer Society developed Camp Sunrise Sidekicks. Sidekicks is a summer camp designed specially for the brothers and sisters of cancer patients. It affords them a chance to develop friendships with other kids in similar circumstances, and to share in the same camp experiences as their sibling.

Children outside of the family can add difficulties to the situation. "Kids are curious, but can also be downright cruel," Noah's mom explains. "If another child asked him what happened to his eye, he'd just put his little head down and tear up. As a parent, I'd come running to the rescue and tell them that he had a boo-boo in his eye, so they had to take it out, and that he will be getting a new one soon."

Noah's mom then met with other mothers who also had children with Retinoblastoma. Noah met other children with prosthetic eyes, like the one he would soon be getting.

His mom tells how, a few days later, he was again approached by kids asking why he didn't have an eye. Just as she was jumping up to go rescue him, he held his head high, and said proudly, "Oh, I had a boo-boo in my eye and the doctor had to take it out, but I'll be getting a new one soon."

Mom reports that his confidence level and self-image magnified after meeting the other kids. She says, "Now, I don't wait for a parent to call me [for advice], I put out the call to them. I answer any questions, and prepare them for what they'll be going through. Then I tell them that, when they're ready, I'd love to have them meet my son, Noah, and see how good he looks with his new eye. It gives them hope and, more importantly, lets them know there is life after cancer."

Katie's mom admits, "You never think it's going to happen to you, or your child." She had to go through it not once, but twice. "The second time around," she says, "all those feelings came right back. 'Oh God, we can't go through this again!' I just wanted to take her place."

With Katie's relapse, they did go through it all over again, but, now age seven, Katie is doing great.

As she rolls her eyes and grins, Katie gives her side of the story, "Ya know, Mom, I could walk out in the street and get hit by a truck tomorrow."

Katie is right. She has faced so many threatening situations in her life that she has unquestionably proven that she is a survivor. What could possibly harm someone who has done the equivalent of leaping tall buildings and stopping speeding locomotives?

Maybe instead of overprotecting, we should allow Katie, and the thousands other childhood cancer survivors like her, to play in traffic, run with scissors, and walk blindfolded with suckers sticking out of their mouths! Right?

Katie's mom thinks not.

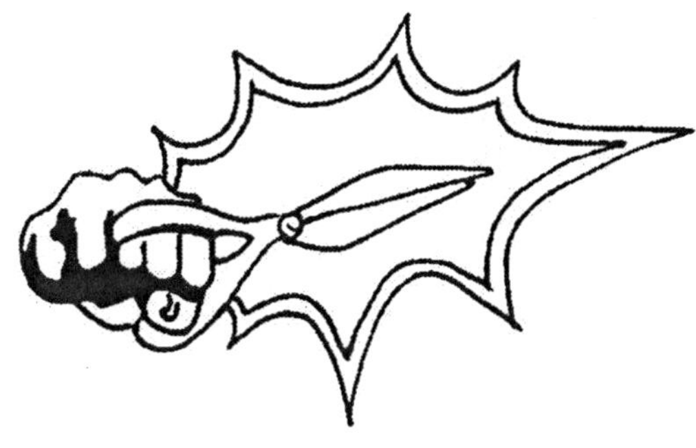

Jell-O War!

Jeoffrey's been hit. He took one in the back. The large green splotch dead center on his previously white t-shirt is a definite clue.

"Direct hit. Woo-hoo!"

Nearby, speckles and blotches of various colors adorn Cami's clothing—red, orange, and a touch of yellow. Jessie seems to be worse off than the both of them. His hair is slicked with gelatin, which is also running down his face. In the distance, a voice rings out, "I can't close my eyes— they're stuck open!"

Welcome to the annual Camp Sunrise Jell-O War!

The competition began shortly after the camp's conception, twenty-some years ago. On a long bus ride to who-knows-where, the campers discussed their individual dislikes of hospital stays. Each had more than their share of pokes, prods, and treatments to recollect, plus their common dislikes of missing school, missing friends, feeling lousy, and not being able to play outside.

One definite similarity arose in their mutual dislike of hospital food—especially, Jell-O. That's right, Jell-O. The mere mention of the stuff set off an entire busload of groans. Already sick, and further nauseated with medications, their food trays usually included the colorful gelatin—sometimes exclusively. Jell-O for breakfast, Jell-O for lunch, Jell-O for dinner—they all agreed, they were burnt out on Jell-O.

"I'd as soon throw it against a wall as eat another bite of Jell-O!" one camper announced.

"Yeah! Jell-O's for throwing, not eating."

They all agreed.

The Camp Director, M, a young volunteer counselor at the time, was present on the bus. Fun loving and open-minded, this sounded good to her. M suggested, "Maybe we should have a Jell-O throwing competition."

Kids being kids, it was quickly suggested that the Jell-O should be thrown at each other. Bingo! A Jell-O fight! And so began the first ever "Jell-O War!"

The Jell-O War has been waged at Camp Sunrise ever since. First, a ridiculous quantity of Jell-O is made and cooled. Jell-O of all colors is cut into cubes and bagged. The closely protected arsenal of gelatin is then transported from the walk-in refrigerator to an undisclosed, remote, and forested site.

Campers and staff volunteers (some wearing protective garbage bag ponchos) are divided into two teams, and everyone is armed with a bag of sticky ammunition. Anticipation runs high while a lengthy explanation of rules, tactics, and regulations is recited.

Rules thoroughly covered, the whistle blows and there is but one stratagem: THROW JELL-O! What follows is complete melee. The only thing clear is that the rules were added only for effect; even the concept of teams quickly disintegrates.

Basically, a person throws, smears, and sticks Jell-O to everyone they find. No one escapes ungelatinized. Jell-O covers your clothing, your hair, and all exposed skin.

Once the war has ended, there are photos to be taken, and then a mass exodus toward the bathhouse and a follow-up battle for the showers.

For over two decades, battles have been fought, clothing has been stained (permanently), and riotous laughter has infected everyone present. It's sick...it's disgusting...and it's the most uniquely healthy war ever waged.

As adults, why can't we solve more of our issues with Jell-O?

(situation:) Rough day at work?
(response:) Throw Jell-O.

(situation:) Someone is speaking poorly of you?
(response:) Throw Jell-O.

(situation:) You get cut off in traffic?
(response:) Throw Jell-O.

On second thought, that's probably not the best idea. But why not handle our problems in a healthy and childlike way, with fun and humor?

Our country loves slogans and catchphrases. Maybe one day the rear bumper of every car driven by an emotionally healthy individual will read:

"When life give you lemons: Throw Jell-O!"

Maybe.

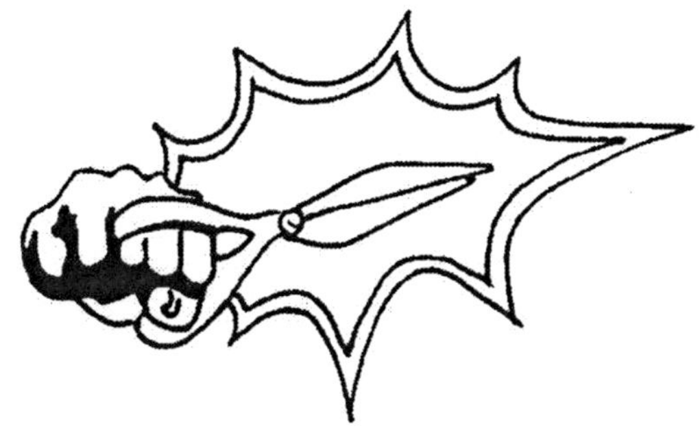

TREES

My friend David can be compared to one of the giant pine trees keeping watch over Camp Sunrise. Observing the top of the tree, it looks vulnerable. It sways in the breeze and, with heavy winds, bends even further. But look lower. Look at the midsection of the tree; its larger branches offer support to the less stable aspects above. Even lower—look at the massive trunk; it's solid and unshakeable.

Some people like to look inside a tree, at its rings. They say that you can not only read the tree's age but can also tell good years from bad. There's a whole book inside each one.

When David first came to camp, he'd been through a rough few months. In March, he'd been diagnosed with a brain tumor and went through three intensive surgeries. The tumor, and subsequent surgeries, left David weak and with extremely poor coordination.

Come July, David was at camp. He was frail, unsteady, a little frightened, and as determined as they come. As a Senior Boy, David's cabin was the furthest from the lodge. The rutted trail weaves uphill and contains plenty of rocks, roots, bushes, and poor footing. David dismissed the idea of bunking in a closer cabin; the cabin at the top of the hill was his, and he'd be staying there. What's more, seemingly oblivious to the fact that he had difficulty standing upright on level ground, David was determined to make the hike on his own.

Weaving up the hill, David would stumble one way or the other, trip on a rock, or fall towards a bush. Each time, one of the other boys was there to catch him. They allowed him to do the hike on his own (he demanded it), but one of them—Ricky, Ralphie, Tyler—was always there to support him in a moment of need.

Each year, David comes back to camp. And, each year, he is stronger and more coordinated. Looking back, David says there is a fine line to determination. It's good to push yourself, but push yourself too far, step over that line, and you get hurt. He also says that that determination enabled him to expand his own limits. He admits that, at times, he got hurt along the way, but says it was worth every bump and bruise.

That first summer, David reminded me of one of those giant pines. Once you looked past his vulnerable exterior—pale, unsteady, and susceptible—you'd see his invincible spirit, sturdy, and impervious. That still holds true.

David certainly is a unique individual, but he's far from being alone. Look around camp and you'll see that same unswerving spark in countless others. In fact, you'll see an entire forest of children and young adults all sharing that same unshakable strength.

If you were to do tree-ring analysis, their stories would each be unique—but their spirit, indistinguishably steadfast.

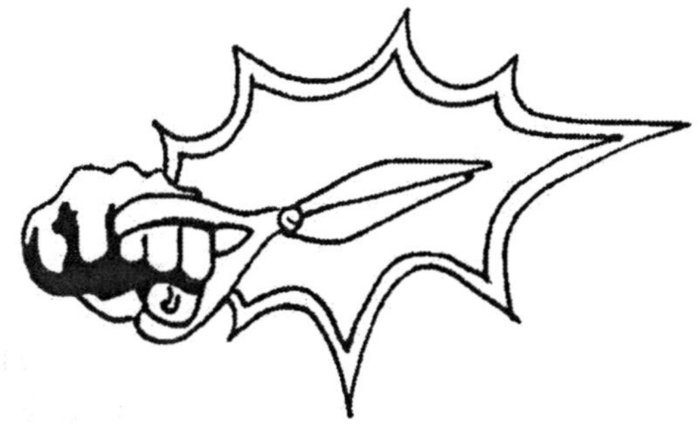

Heather & Himmelman

I'd like to tell you about my friend Heather. She's five-foot-two, ninety-eight pounds, and has the strength of 10,000 men. But first, let me tell you about Peter Himmelman. He's an incredible artist, and an amazing person. But this isn't about him; this is about a song.

Peter put out a song about a woman he'd met. You've probably heard it on the radio. Although the lyrics seem a bit odd—***I was speaking to you with my voice / you were talkin' to me by choosing letters with your eyebrow***—I knew it was powerful stuff.

Later, I had the good fortune to see Pete in concert. Prior to playing the song, he told the crowd how his uncle had wanted him to meet a girl who was a fan of his music. Upon entering her home, he discovered that she was a quadriplegic, paralyzed, and wheelchair bound. Her only way of communicating with the outside world was via computer. Things were rigged up so she could push buttons on a keyboard using her eyebrow, the only part of her body she had control over. It turns out the lyrics to the song are, in fact, quite literal.

Her positive outlook on life, and her accomplishments, in the face of her obvious obstacles, moved Peter. At the same time, he explained, he felt self-conscious and that he owed her an apology for the days of his own life he had let slide right through his hands. Peter Himmelman used his own abilities to put it down in song, dubbing her, "The Woman with the Strength of 10,000 Men."

That's powerful stuff.

But I'm not here to talk about a song; I'm here to talk about my friend, Heather.

At age 10, Heather underwent brain surgery to remove a cancerous tumor. The removal of the tumor stunted her growth and left her weak, unsteady, and with poor vision. If you were to ask Heather, she would tell you she didn't see too well after dark. Then she would take your arm so you could help guide her past obstacles in the road. I liked that.

Actually, Heather was legally blind and couldn't see well even in daylight. But she made do, never complaining. What little eyesight she had was rapidly deserting her, so she decided to learn brail. She told me that her instructor would get upset with her for peeking while she practiced. She laughed as she told it, "Hey, as long as my eyes work a little, I may as well use them, right?"

Heather was like that.

Heather taught me a lot about not taking things for granted. She taught me that when problems, or obstacles, hinder my path, not to let them get me down.

I miss Heather.

I cried when I heard of her passing. I even cried before I heard of her passing; I guess it's one of those things you just sense.

Heather isn't here any more. I can't call her, or send her an e-mail. We don't sit on a picnic table and talk, and she doesn't take my arm when it's getting dark. I miss that.

Heather is still with me though. She hasn't abandoned me, and wouldn't. Daily, Heather consoles me with comfort and direction. She guides me around the obstacles in the road, and reminds me, "Don't let it get you down; there's no time to waste on such things."

Heather is my friend. She's the woman with the strength of 10,000 men.

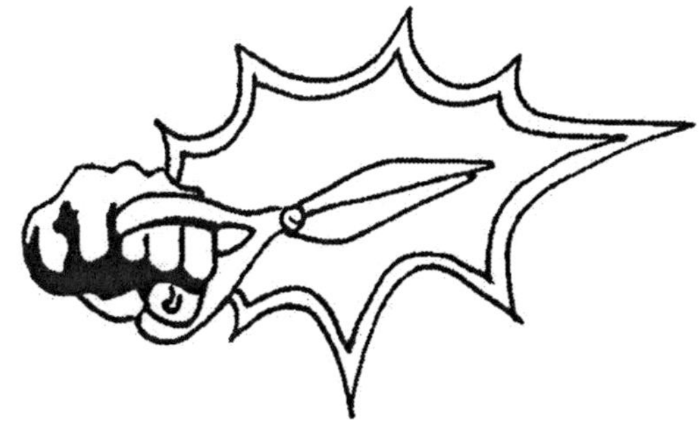

"The THING?"

"Wow, 'The THING?'!"
"'The THING?' What's 'The THING?'?"
"You know...'The THING?'"
"Oh."
"I've seen it."
"You've seen 'The THING?'"
"Well, no...but I think my dad has."
"But what is it?"
"It's just 'The THING?'"
"But, really, what is it?"
"It's, ummmmm... you know, 'The THING?'"

My favorite t-shirt sparked a conversation between kids, and, at their insistence, allowed me to tell the story of America's most purposefully vague tourist attraction.

You've might have seen the billboards. How could you miss them? Bright yellow billboards with bold blue printing—miles and miles of billboard, after billboard, after billboard—they are undoubtedly intriguing, and I was helpless to their power.

"The Mystery of the Desert!"
Moccasins...
Rattlesnake Heads...

Blankets...
Wind Chimes...
"The THING?"

It is one of life's great mysteries, an enigma, and I was about to find it out once and for all.

The parking lot was full of automobiles, and my mind full of questions. Just what is "The THING?"? Why haven't I made it here previously? Why is there a Dairy Queen in the same building? And, why is everything here punctuated with either an exclamation point or a question mark?

Strange!

As I walked toward the entrance it was impossible not to notice the semi-dazed tourists exiting the building, obviously deep in their own thoughts. I couldn't help but ask myself, *does "The THING?" turn you into a zombie-tourist with its' penetrating death-beam eyes?*

I wondered.

In the curio shop I found a stuffed armadillo on its back hugging a Lone-Star beer bottle. There was a Jack-a-lope, t-shirts, key-chains, and bumper stickers. Even a rattlesnake head with fangs bared, wearing a mop-top toupee' and funky dangling earrings, all atop a body resembling a tiny wooly-mammoth cum fluffy-ferret-thing. They had it all. Classic curio-crapola!

The man behind the counter was ancient and had a tattered straw hat to match. Was he "The THINGS?" manager? I didn't know, but handed over my dollar.

With my ticket stub in hand, and a strange mix of curiosity, excitement, and trepidation, I approached the cavernous entrance to meet "The THING?"

The door anti-climactically led out back, to a courtyard lined with corrugated steel sheds. Feeling like Fred from Scooby-Doo, I followed the size forty-four yellow footprints on the sidewalk. The jumbo prints lead me into the first structure. Finally, the lair of "The THING?".

Actually, no. It was not the highly anticipated lair of "The THING?," but an old shed full of junk...er, antiques. (O-kay, "antique-junk" would be more accurate.) They toyed with my already elevated emotions by hiking me through that and another shed littered with peculiar riff-raff. O-kay, enough hokey build-up, I was ready to see "The THING?" As I entered the third shed I could tell it was the one I'd been waiting for. A large sign read, "'The THING?'—What is it?"

Directly beneath the sign was a large, heavily battered, wooden case. I held my breath as I approached. There it was. Underneath the glass, smudged by fifty years of tourist fingerprints, was...well... "The THING?" Yes, "The THING?!"

I was speechless.

Really, speechless...

The thing about "The THING?" is...well, it's kind of hard to explain. Let's just say that certain questions arise. Big, awkward, hard-to-get-your-mind-around questions.

Questions like:
"Where d'ya think it came from?"
"How'd it get here?"
"Is it for real?"
"Whad'ya think they feed it?"
"Is that what I think it is?"
"Do you think there are more 'The THINGS?'?"
And then:
"How many people, like myself, do you think pay a dollar to see "The THING?" each day?"
"How many dollars would that be in a year?"
"If 'The THING?' has been here for fifty years, isn't that a whole lot of money?"

"Does that mean that 'The THING?' is rich?"
"Does 'The THING?' have a bank account?"
"Do we leave now?"
"Anyone for a Peanut Buster Parfait?"

The exit lead right back to the curio shop. Ah, safety and sanity at last! (Odd that a place selling stuffed armadillos gave me a secure feeling, but it did.) I stumbled my way back to the parking lot, silent, and a bit dazed. I was now one of the zombie-tourists.

Unanswered questions continued to rattle around in my brain. Odd, disturbing, kinda creepy, and disenchanting questions. "Was that...? But... Whooooooa!"

In hindsight, it's important to pick up a commemorative t-shirt and key-chain at the same time you pay your admission fee—prior to entering. Fortunately, I had. Otherwise, fuzzyheaded as I was, I would have risked not thinking clearly enough to purchase some memorabilic proof of the visit. That would have been an unfortunate faux pas, as I find great satisfaction in proudly wearing my t-shirt and encouraging everyone to rush off and experience "The THING?" for themselves.

Really, it's an experience you won't regret...er, forget... or, uh... nevermind.

Like "The THING?," there are a lot of unknowns, mysteries, and conundrums around. Life is full of them.

"Why are we here?"
"What is the meaning of life?"
"What *is* that slimy stuff around a block of Spam?"
"What's it all about?"

Sometimes it seems we just don't get it—whatever "it" is.

Many of us get so tied up in the rush of our day-to-day activities that we go for entire days, weeks, without taking a moment to truly appreciate life.

Thornton Wilder wrote about it back in 1938. He said that we move about in a cloud of ignorance and blindness, missing out on life even as we live it. We trample on feelings, spend and waste time as if we have a million years. We just don't get it.

Some say that saints and poets get it. They then attempt to give the rest of us a glimpse of the big picture. Sometimes they succeed. Others say that as children we get it, but begin to forget "it" as we age.

I don't know.

This is often true of a child who has been through cancer. They've been there, dealt with it first hand, and have an understanding beyond anything we could ever imagine. Having been there provides them with an acquired wisdom, knowledge of the big picture, an ability to look past the little things and fully realize life while they live it.

It's wisdom beyond their years, learned from the greatest guru of all—LIFE.

Society puts forth a lot of smoke screens that distort our vision—prefab definitions of success, what is important, what's real. Unfortunately, it often isn't until we get smacked in the head by a real crisis that we back up, focus, and get a more realistic perspective on things.

James Joyce likened it to what he called "the whispers and the screams." We all receive little whispers on a regular basis, they attempt to keep us on track. We need to acknowledge those whispers and do something in response. Other times, the screams come. Sometimes it takes a shocking, life-threatening scream to wake us up. Cancer is one such scream and often affords people another perspective. It gives us a chance to reevaluate what is important in life and what it is all about.

It's a chance to "get it."

Aubrie had cancer; she's been there. She'll tell you, "You shouldn't wait for tragedy to happen to start appreciating life."

Aubrie had a non-Hodgkin's lymphoma and endured some difficult times, including radiation and chemotherapy. How does she feel about her experience with cancer? "All in all," she says, "it has definitely been a positive experience, and I wouldn't take it back for anything."

The same sentiment is echoed by countless other cancer survivors. Cancer may have threatened their lives, but it also gave them a whole new perspective, which enhanced their lives in degrees without parallel.

Harvey says, "We're all put on earth for a reason." He had acute lymphocytic leukemia as a young child and has since celebrated his tenth anniversary since remission. Harvey has remained true to his end of the bargain. "I owe a lot to a lot of people," he says, "so I try to pay some of it back. It's in my contract."

Not only has Harvey been attending oncology camps for more than twenty years—first as a camper, and now a counselor—he works with a school system assisting underprivileged children with their needs. Harvey attributes his drive and dedication to his cancer experience early in life.

I certainly would not wish cancer on anyone, but possibly—after the poking and prodding, tears and fears have subsided—we could reap benefits from the experience. Perhaps we would treat each other better. Maybe we would quit wasting days and better appreciate each moment. Maybe we'd have a more loving and tolerant society.

Maybe.

Wouldn't it be infinitely better if we could learn our lessons by the example of others? Why go through the horrors when we have others that have already been there. Truly benevolent individuals who offer their knowledge openly, as witnessed by the way they live their lives. Like the children of Camp Sunrise, these are the ones with the treasures of a unique perspective.

They are the ones that get it.

Maybe the lesson we need to learn from these young sages involves our need to simplify. To liberate ourselves from all the "isms" and "ologies" that society shackles us with. Possibly the lesson is to live each moment for what it is—a specific, unique, and precious fragment of time. If we aren't able to appreciate this moment, right now, can we really appreciate any moment, ever? Perhaps we shouldn't wait until things slow down at the office, or until we have more time, or until the weekend, or until tomorrow.

Maybe the message these modern day masters of wisdom bring us is not to put things off until after dinner, or after awhile, or until anytime later, but to enjoy each moment in the now. Inhale it, absorb it, make it our own.

If we don't appreciate this moment, right now, we lose it. We lose the moment, we lose the now, we lose the chance to appreciate its beauty. Sure, there'll be other moments to appreciate later—down the road when we have more time—but our only opportunity to experience *this* moment, is now.

Camper David does a good job of summing up that message. He says, "Don't wait. Enjoy life now—right now!"

Bob Wallace

David is right. It's about adding life to our days—every, every day.

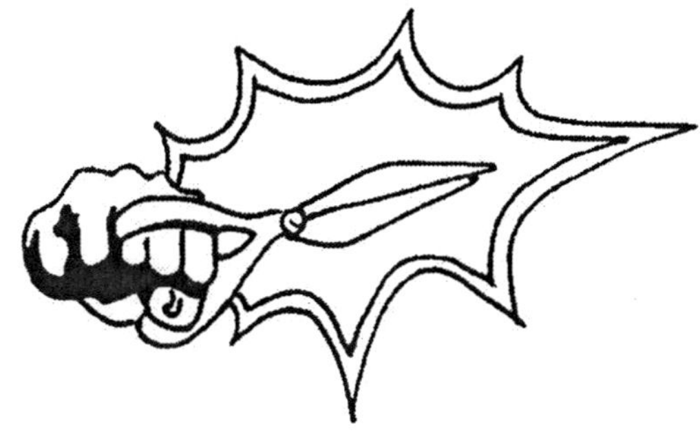

Dictionaries and Daredevils

To find the official definition of **"superhero,"** I thought I'd go to the dictionary. Not just any dictionary, The Compact Oxford English Dictionary (New Edition). It's like the Big Kahuna of all dictionaries. It's as complete as they come, and only really smart people own them, or would want to. I borrowed the book (duh!), having decided it would be the place to go for a definitive definition of the word **"superhero."**

What I envisioned was a concise definition, full of clarity. I was sadly mistaken. The word **"superhero"** was not in the book.

Flashing back to grade school, I knew just what to do. I would look up the root-word **"super"** and then the...uh, not-so-root-word **"hero."** (O-kay, so I don't remember that much from grade school.)

Success! But it was no easy task.

First, let me tell you a little more about The Compact Oxford English Dictionary (New Edition). In the front of the book it tells us that the compact edition contains the entire text, unaltered in all essentials, of the original twelve-volume set. Twelve volumes! Plus, it contains the complete text of a four-volume supplement to the original set. Whew!

Bottom line, it's sixteen books squeezed into one massive volume. It weighs eighteen pounds, is the cause of many intellectual hernias, and comes with a high-tech magnifying glass the size of a full-grown otter's head. The glass does have truly amazing optical qualities, (a grasshopper wouldn't stand a chance under one of these babies!), which is vital, because the words are so ridiculously small that, without the magnifier, it would require superhuman vision to look up the word "**superhuman**."

The assorted definitions of the word "**super**" permeated two-thirds of one gigantic page. Let's do the math. The book was shrunk from sixteen volumes to one, so, we can suppose, the plethora of definitions for the word "**super**" would take up about eight pages in the full-sized book. (Is it just me, or does this seem a little excessive?) Eight pages! That's a lot of reading. Especially when you consider that we both knew basically what the word meant before looking it up.

For your own protection, allow me to paraphrase the definition. The prefix "**super**" is used to denote a person, animal, or thing that markedly exceeds all others, or the generality, of its class. (Whatever...) The suffix "**hero**" refers to a man or woman who exhibits extraordinary bravery, firmness, fortitude, or greatness of soul, in any course of action; a man or woman admired and venerated for his or her achievements and noble qualities.

There it is, clear as mud.

Superhero: To many, a Speedo-wearing caped crusader may come to mind. To me, Drew comes to mind. Also Alysssa, and Megan, and Cody come to mind. There's also Justin, and Michael, and Kyle, and Ryan, and Leonard, and Andrea, and Donny, and Britannie, and Lacey, and Gian, and Lani, and Kimberly, and Mathew, and Alexander, and Cortney, and Bridgett, and Matt, and Shane, and Keenan, and

Kyle, and Jeffery, and Marquis, and Brittany, and RaySean, and David, and Marina, and Eric, and Meghan, and Shelby, and Jacob, and Mariah, and Robby, and Celina, and Dustin, and Adam, and Mikayla, and Tanya, and Sasha, and Alex, and Abriel, and Ricky, and Joshua, and Jairess, and Tyler, and Matt, and Amanda, and Amy, and Beth, and Lorissa, and Killian, and Kelsey, and Savanna, and Toria, and Saraswati, and Sarah, and Kyle, and Katie, and Cheyenne, and Liz, and Serena, and David, and Mathew, and Bobby, and Sabrina, and Alyssa, and Luzelena, and Carlos, and Ryan, and Justin, and Visha, and Nathan, and Kathy, and Tim, and Megan, and Meghann, and Amber, and Devon, and Jesse, and Jimmy, and Michael, and Casey, and Dakota, and Kim, and Kristin, and Sonja, and Brandyn, and Tiffany, and Ashley, and Stevie, and Daniel, and Chad, and Antonita, and Tyler, and Rafael, and Mark, and Derek, and Nichole, and Katie, and Christopher, and Jason, and Megan, and Robert, and Brittnee, and Geoffrey, and Eron, and Cassandra, and Paula, and Stephenie, and Kalyn, and Sarah, and Heather, and Dylan, and Jared, and Danielle, and Steven, and Leah, and Cami, and Susan, and William, and Justin, and Randi, and Evan, and Cindy, and Tobin, and James, and Bryant, and so many, many more.

The definition fits each of these kids to a "**t**." Each of them far exceeds the general grouping of individuals, in that they've been through so much. They've endured inconceivable hardship, yet come out undaunted. That's pretty super. While battling cancer they each exhibited extraordinary bravery and fortitude. As for greatness of soul, they are masters. One can't help but admire and respect these pint-sized superheroes for the miraculous things they have achieved, and for their countless noble qualities.

Like I said, to a "**t**."

Let me tell you about the tiniest superhero I know. No, it's not the citizens of the miniature city of Kandor who got shrunk and placed in a bottle by the evil genius Braniac. It's MJ.

At seventeen months, MJ was diagnosed with A.L.L., acute lymphocytic leukemia. Unlike the citizens of Kandor, MJ will not be contained. She went through some tough months during chemotherapy and is on a maintenance routine now.

MJ is now an active two-year-old, and I recently witnessed her first horseback ride. Soon, MJ will be living out a very normal childhood; playing Pretty, Pretty Princess, celebrating birthdays, and growing into a beautiful super-heroine.

One day she'll probably blush when reading this, scarcely realizing what an amazing girl she really is.

As I glance across the lodge, I see the Epoxy Biker riding wheelies with Shopping Diva on the back of his bike, her red hair flowing in the breeze. The Red Vine Ranger is doing rope tricks with her licorice lasso, while the Atomic Punk wails through a laser-shooting guitar solo. Elsewhere, Monkey Fist is defending the world from a particularly dangerous junior girl, while Beastie Boy howls in delight.

Watching the mayhem, I am truly in awe of each and every one of them. Protected by the "Justice League of Camp Sunrise," I've never felt more secure in the thought that the earth will always be safe, beautiful, and anything but boring.

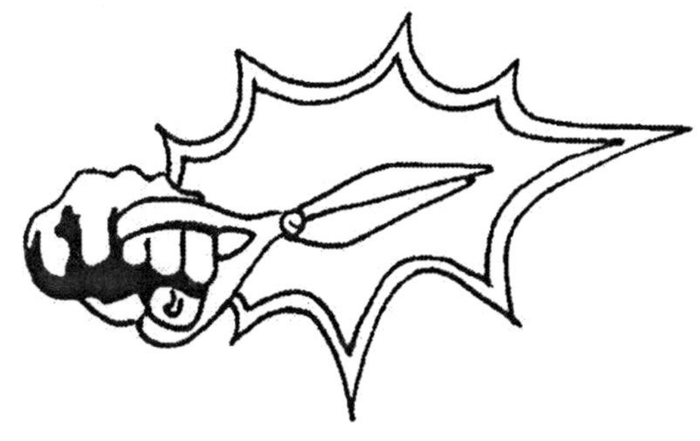

Memories: (Dance Mix)

This summer's theme at Camp Sunrise is "National Holidays." Today is "Milk Day." It's some twisted emulation of "M.L.K." day. (Add an "I" and you have "MILK"—go figure.) We've been playing milk-related games all afternoon, and still sport the permanent milk mustaches painted on our upper lips first thing this morning.

Robby, wearing his long white, "got milk?" t-shirt, milk ball-cap, and bare feet, is competitively attempting to pick marbles out of a large vat of sour cream using only his toes. Robby was hesitant at first, and protested loudly, but now his laughter is louder yet. The sour cream is cold, stinky, and feels...well, pretty much how you'd imagine a vat of sour cream to feel to your toes. Yuck!

Robby, with an uncanny display of toe-to-eye coordination, salvages five marbles from the gooey mess in the time allotted. To Robby, this is some real fun. To the rest of us, it's a snapshot in time.

* * *

It's the first day of Yoga Class and my buddy Mathew is enrolled. (Who it was that convinced him to sign up for yoga is uncertain. At least nothing has been proven.) The yoga instructor, Linda, is a tall, dynamic blonde in her first year of law school. Mathew is a bit shorter, also blonde, and every bit as dynamic, as he experiences his first ever yoga class. Linda is unsure how he will fit in with the class. Mathew is unsure the class is what he was looking for. Both are willing to give it a go.

Moments later, emanating from the cabin, we hear, "Hey, this isn't Kung Fu!"

Words to warm the heart.

* * *

The camp tree house? Oh, that. It's a much talked about yet rarely witnessed monstrosity. The tree house, like Snipe hunting and Kevin, the tree house founder, is a camp legend.

Often standing silently in the background, Kevin is a self-proclaimed Idea Man. Need a new game? How about "Butt-Flap Dodge-Ball/Velcro Loincloth." (Does it have a real name, Kevin?) Need an all-camp activity? Let's build an ice cream sundae on top of our best friend's head from a good twelve feet above. Not weird enough for you? How about we dip pancakes in chocolate pudding and then...well, you get the idea. Kevin has masterminded so many games and activities that we finally just gave him his own day—"Kevin's Day." (If attending, plan on having a lot of fun, but, please, wear disposable clothes!)

The tree house seemed like a great idea—a few tools, some lumber, and there's no lack of trees— what could be easier. Employing the Senior Boys to carry all tools and materials up the mountain showed good planning. The number of hours required to build the tree house of Kevin's imagination exceeded the plan, but it was completed.

Imagine, if you can, a lumbering camouflaged box levitating between four trees and you'll get an idea—kind of. In actuality, like Stonehenge and the Grecian Parthenon, it's an architectural masterpiece you really have to experience for yourself.

Unfortunately, even if you know where the behemoth resides, you still have to cross the creek and climb the mountain. Even then, you probably won't see it until it's suddenly looming over your head. The tree house has been viewed by few, and fewer yet have reclined in its roomy interior. But many talk about it, hence, its legendary appeal.

For years the tree house has withstood snow, rain, wind, and weather of all types. Yet it stands...er, hangs as a tribute to Camp Sunrise ingenuity and Idea Men everywhere.

* * *

Waking the morning after the Formal Dinner and Dance, the mirror reveals a face full of blue ink resembling the battle scene from Braveheart. (That was the intention last night, anyway.) As you reach for the soap, you vaguely recall not being able to find the face paints and being assured by the entire Ladybug cabin that blue permanent marker would be a fine substitute.

(Author's note: It's been my experience that eight-year-old girls are more than happy to solve any and all of your makeup problems.)

Back to the mirror. Let's see...it's Saturday now, and, in the real world, you need to be at work Monday morning. Let's hope this works.

It doesn't.

"Cold cream," Shelby suggests, "that'll take it off."

It doesn't.

A frantic ransacking of the kitchen supply cabinets produces a harsh detergent and Brillo pads. These do work, but their effectiveness relies on removing several layers of skin along with the ink. We'll reserve this as a last resort.

Where better than camp to find someone with a solution to such issues? And who better to go to then Barb, ACS's head of Childhood Development. If anyone, she will know just what to do.

Having grown up with older siblings of your own, Barb's solution sounds more than a little suspicious, and, having fallen prey to her practical jokes in the past, you are skeptical. But, desperate times call for desperate measures, so you follow her instructions.

1) add additional quantities of dry-erase marker over top of the permanent marker...
2) let dry...
3) simply, wash the whole mess off with soap and water.

Miracles of miracles, Barb was not pulling your leg, and you are
de-Bravehearted without any difficulty at all.
Camp knowledge runs deep!

* * *

When a nine-year-old camper immediately asks if you know what **antidisestablishmentarianism** is, you should know you are in trouble. Later—after getting the entire cabin tucked in their sleeping bags, relatively quiet, and flashlights off—when another child asks, "So are you guys going out on the front porch to talk?" you *definitely* should have a clue.

But, you don't. "Yes, I believe we will," Dustin replies.

It's the camp's Winter Retreat and it is cold outside. It's one a.m. when you and the other counselors—having caught up on what's going on in each other's lives, laughed over campers' activities, and gotten chilled to the bone—decide to turn in to your own sleeping bags. This is where the problem arises. The doorknob doesn't turn. Ben checks the rear of the cabin and finds that the back door is also locked.

"O-kay, funny prank, you got us guys," Stumpy yells. "Now let us in."

In unison you beat on the door and rap on the windows, but none of the kids stir. This continues for some time, with absolutely no response from the exhausted nine-year-olds inside. Finally, chilled beyond the bone, Ben manages to find an unlocked window. He removes the screen, and climbs through.

Just to confirm that no one is faking sleep, Dustin sets off the remote control fart-machine a couple of times. (It's a proven fact: No matter how devious a kid is, no boy can resist giggling at flatulence.) There is not so much as a peep out of the kids. Obviously, they are truly asleep.

"No one else needs to know about this, right?" Stumpy whispers.

"Right," says Ben. "What happens on the porch, stays on the porch." Each of you agrees, and turns in.

The next morning, on the way to the lodge, each of you is greeted with smirks and giggles. After breakfast, Mike pauses the announcements and recaps the entire event over the P.A. system for everyone's enjoyment.

It just goes to show, there are no secrets at camp.

* * *

My friend Derrick just showed me a card trick. Derrick—burly, round faced, and handsome—seems to have traded in his favorite Scooby-Doo t-shirt for a button-up dress shirt this year. He looks sharp and, this time, the card trick works perfectly. Over the past couple years I've seen the trick maybe a dozen times. Sometimes it works, sometimes it doesn't.

"Want to know how I did it?" he asks.

"No, Derrick, some things are best left unexplained. Just let me enjoy the magic of the unknown."

"Want me to do it again?"

"Sure, Derrick. One more time."

Derrick and I shared a table at the Formal Dinner once—kind of a double-date thing. He wore his best shirt, dress pants, shiny shoes, and a lot of cheap aftershave. (I always bring plenty to share for the occasion). Me? I believe I was dressed as a Hawaiian shark.

I was encouraging Derrick to be extra polite, carry his date's tray, get her an extra glass of milk, things like that. Before long, he gritted his teeth and told me, "How about this. You mind your date's business, and I'll mind mine."

When you think about it, those are pretty good words of wisdom. In the future I'll try to heed his advice.

* * *

Supplies: One bucket; a mop wringer; one plastic serving spoon; duct tape; and a healthy dose of nine-year-old ingenuity.

Result: One fully functional catapult.

Usage: Launching marshmallows off the porch toward a mob of hyper kids with lofty intentions of catching them in their mouths.

Final score: Rhinos win, with a total of 250 points.

* * *

If you've ever been "Trucked," you won't likely forget it. And then again...you might.

"Trucking" is purely an Camp Sunrise thing. It's kind of a rights-of-passage if you will, and, therefore, I'm not permitted to talk about it.

Unless, of course, you know the secret handshake.

* * *

<u>21 Things the Kids Taught Me:</u>

1) Every bone marrow aspiration hurts as much as the one before. You will never get used to them.
2) Hair grows back.
3) You can find humor in anything.
4) Valuable experiences and important lessons can really suck sometimes.
5)Singing and dancing, even out-of-key and poorly, are good for you. (Correction: *especially* out-of-key and poorly.)
6) Sometimes things that taste bad are good for you. (and vice-versa).
7) A hospital is just a place to visit.
8) Things do get better.
9) A physical handicap can be worn like a medal of honor.
10) You can learn a lot from looking back, and you can create anything looking forward.
11) You can make a hat out of almost anything.
12) Cancer sucks.
13) You're not alone.
14) Being old doesn't make you wise, and being young doesn't mean you haven't experienced life.

15) Throwing food can be healthy.
16) The unknown can be terrifying, or exciting. It's your choice.
17) When playing Pictionary, if you don't know what the thing is, you can still draw stuff.
18) Fashion accessories made with food items should always include an expiration date.
19) Girls can be cool, and boys aren't *always* disgusting.
20) If you feel like having another cookie, have another cookie.
21) Live life—every, every day!

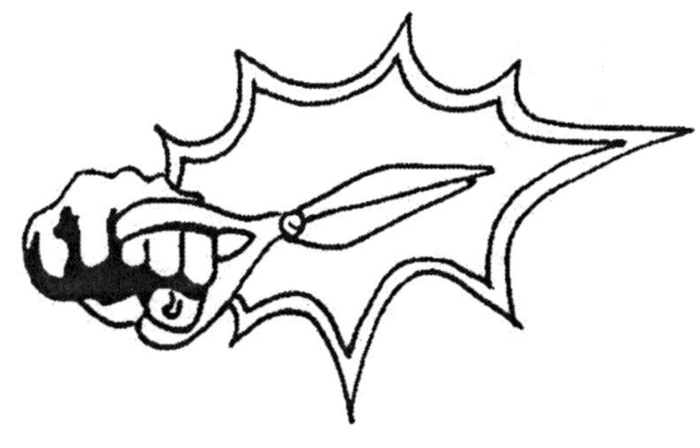

MJA & BBP

"Look! It's Bumblebee Planet!"

I didn't have any idea what little Caroline was talking about, but her enthusiasm was contagious and I soon found myself every bit as excited as she.

"Bumblebee Planet? No way!" I cried.

"Yes, Bumblebee Planet—see?"

I did see, but didn't know what it was I was seeing. It looked like tiny overlapping circles on her hand. Was it a birthmark? ink? a smudge of dirt?—I didn't know.

"Wow," I said, "where'd you get that, Caroline?"

"It was just there," she explained matter-of-fact, "Michael put it there."

"Michael? Your brother Michael?"

"Yes, he left it there for me—see?"

As I meticulously inspected her beauty mark, my thoughts were on her brother. Michael was one of those kids who have a profound impact on the world. Let me tell you his story:

Michael J. Arias came into this world blue-eyed and raring to go. His parents were obviously proud of their son, and gave him as much love as any child has received. Michael was as happy, exuberant, and charismatic as they come. None could deny the allure of the energetic child with the bright blue eyes.

Things were ideal at the Arias home, and no family was more content. Sadly, that was all to change.

When Michael was three, he was diagnosed with cancer. It was a stage IV neuroblastoma—a cancer of the sympathetic nervous system, which originated in his adrenal gland and spread to his bone marrow, ribs, legs, and spine—the prognosis was poor. Michael's family took the news as well as could be expected, and set out to do everything possible to return their son to good health.

At just three years of age, Michael underwent a full treatment of chemotherapy, a lot for a child to endure. Still, Michael remained upbeat.

While undergoing that first round of chemotherapy, Michael had a long stay in the hospital. One day, feeling well enough to spend some time in the Child Life Room, he joined the other children in making bumblebees out of construction paper.

His bumblebee was hung from his IV pole.

Michael woke up the next morning excited to tell his mother of a place where he had traveled. A place where there were no doctors, no needles, no pills, and no ouches—a place he called Bumblebee Planet.

Michael would draw pictures of Bumblebee Planet, and the rocket ship he used to get there. He loved his excursions to Bumblebee Planet, the one place where he never had a worry. The rocket Michael traveled in had four windows—one for him; one for Blakin, a little girl he had become friends with in the hospital; and a window each for his imaginary friends, Johnny and Hockey. Michael shared many pictures and stories of their adventures to Bumblebee Planet.

One day, his mother noticed an addition to his rocket ship.

"Who is the fifth window for?" she asked.

With bright eyes, Michael responded, "It's for you. Would you like to go to Bumblebee Planet with us?"

His mother was delighted, and shared in a wonderful voyage to her son's tiny planet. On the outing she learned that Bumblebee Planet was even smaller than she realized. So tiny, in fact, that there was only enough room for a Home Depot, a Toys-R-Us, the four pioneers, and her.

From then on Michael would occasionally invite someone to sit at the fifth window. His dad, one of his doctors, and his grandma were all honored to make the trip. Bumblebee Planet became a huge thing to the entire family, and it was a wonderful coping mechanism for difficult times.

That summer, Michael attended the Summer Fun Day Camp, put on by the American Cancer Society. Being only three when diagnosed, he had no peer group outside of the hospital and Day Camp provided him his own set of friends. Soon he began collecting friends of all ages. Michael loved Day Camp, and the Airus family was hopeful.

The cancer, and subsequent treatment, played havoc on Michael's tiny body, yet he fought valiantly. More than once he hit bottom, his white blood cells and immune system were nearly nonexistent, and the doctors were not optimistic. More than once, Michael bounced back, and fears were lessened.

Through this time, Michael continued to go to Day Camp; he insisted upon it. Nurse Margaret remembers, "We'd receive news that Michael wasn't doing well, and then, low-and-behold, he'd show up back at Day Camp. He was weak and hairless, but still raring to go!"

Many were the days that Michael would insist on going to Day Camp, but would pass-out, exhausted, on the ride over and would sleep through the whole morning. The next day, he'd be just as determined, and would do it all over again.

Being too sick to attend the ACS Balloon Festival, one of the pilots volunteered to come to his home and take him for a ride. Michael, his father, and the pilot flew high above the neighborhood and right over his own backyard.

Thinking it would be the most incredible thing to Michael, his parents were surprised to see a disappointed look on his face following the ride. "What's wrong," his mom asked, "didn't you like the balloon ride?"

"Yeah, it was nice," he said. Then, with a puzzled look, he asked, "But why was Dad taking me up there?"

"Well, we thought you would find it fun," she responded.

"Oh...o-kay," Michael said. "It was fine."

Curious, his mother asked, "Why did you think he was taking you up in the balloon?"

Michael responded casually, "I thought dad was taking me to heaven."

Michael's cancer relapsed, and he had to go back into treatment. Michael battled heroically, but his body continued to do poorly. When the usual avenues of treatment were exhausted, far from giving up, Michael's parents took him to California for additional treatment involving new drugs and protocols still considered experimental.

Trying to keep things as normal as possible for the family, his parents would refer to the frequent trips to the coast as vacations, and made sure that

Michael and his younger brother and sister got to see the sights and have some fun. Michael's favorite activity was going to the aquarium to watch the sharks.

Michael touched many lives during this difficult time in his own. While receiving treatment at USC, a fraternity hosting a charity dance marathon for the Miracle Network invited him to join them. Feeling lousy, yet still gregarious, Michael agreed to go.

Later, through one of the frat brothers, Michael was introduced to Rob Perelka, who played for the 1995 World Champion Arizona Rattlers. He was immediately enamored by the little boy's charm.

While sitting on Rob's lap, Michael asked, "What's that?" pointing to the huge ring on his finger.

"That's my championship ring," he responded, letting Michael place the ring on his own tiny finger.

"Hey look," Michael exclaimed, "I'm a champion too!"

"That you are," Rob replied. "You're a champion in more ways than you'll ever know!"

That moment blossomed into the "Champion Water Program"— a retail bottled water program that donates a percentage of its proceeds to "Every Kid Counts," a charity raising money to help families in need. Michael was the "Champion of the Year" and had his picture on the side of every bottle. Later, the program joined forces with Phoenix Children's Hospital, and now benefits their cancer center, as well.

There is also a cancer research lab at Arizona State University bearing Michael's name. And, at the Long Beach Aquarium, you'll find a plaque on one of the shark cages with his name and one of his favorite sayings, "Don't get caught in the dark, shark."

Michael and his family battled his cancer for three years, at which time, Michael J. Arias passed away. We lost a truly wonderful child, but not before making his mark on the world. His enchanting charisma exponentially touched the lives of so many people—many he never actually met.

Michael is a testament to it not being the length of time you spend on earth, but the quality, that matters.

One day in September, a month prior to his death, Michael had been feeling a little stronger and was concentrating on drawing pictures—stacks and stacks of pictures. His mother asked him why he was working so hard.

"It's so you won't be too lonely when I'm gone," he told her.

Michael's understanding of his own condition was difficult for his mother to handle. A couple days later he was again feeling pretty good. Enjoying his cheer, his mom asked, "What are you so happy about today?"

"I'm excited about the baby," he told her.

"What baby?"

"Our baby," he replied, barely looking up.

Perplexed, his mother responded, "But we're not having a baby."

"Yes we are," he beamed.

"Now, why would you say that?" she asked.

"God told me," was his matter-of-fact response. "God said that you're going to have a baby girl and that we should name her Caroline."

In November, a month after his death, Michael's mother was taken aback when the doctor told her that, indeed, she was pregnant. The parents chose not to find out the baby's gender in advance, but, the following April, a healthy baby girl was born, blue-eyed and raring to go.

There was no question as to her name; her big brother had named her many months prior. Michelle was then chosen as Caroline's middle name—after her brother.

Caroline's features, mannerisms, and baby photos are a mirror of her older brother's. She is as happy, exuberant, and charismatic as they come, and none will deny the allure of this energetic child with the bright blue eyes.

Caroline does have one very distinguishing feature, though. Her little hand displays a birthmark of tiny overlapping circles, a reminder of good times in a place where there's no ouches and no worries— Bumblebee Planet.

She wears it like a badge of honor, and is more than happy to share it with all of us. "Look! It's Bumblebee Planet!"

Caroline is not seen as a replacement for Michael, but she does help make up for some of the loss. Her mother looks forward to the day when her daughter will be old enough to learn all about her amazing big brother, and how he touched so many lives.

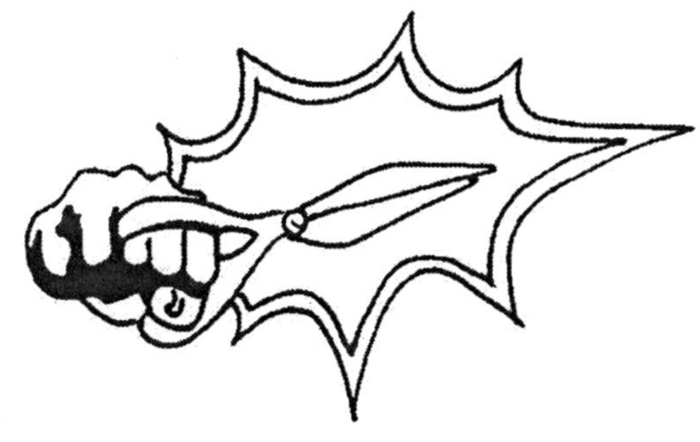

Flatulence

"Shhhhhhh...did you hear that?"
"Hear what?"
"-toot-"
"Hee, hee, hee."
"Hey Jimmy, pull my finger."
"—rrrrrrrrrriiiiiiip—"
"Ha, ha, ha, ha, ha!"
"So whatcha eattin' under there?"
"Under where?"
"Whoa, ho, ho, ho, ho!"
"Wheew! Who cut the cheese?"
"Wasn't me..."
"Or me..."
"Silent, but deadly!"
"Blame it on the dog."
"Did someone say, 'Pass the gas?' Coming up..."
"That's it, no more refried beans for any of you!"

Boys are a disgusting lot, every last one of them. Now, I've never farted myself, but I've certainly experienced them from the vantage point of an innocent bystander. (An olfactory spectator, if you will.) How is it kids, boys in particular, can take a perfectly healthy thing like gas and turn it into such juvenile humor? Potty humor, that's what it is.

Gas is good... Gas is healthy... And wholesome... Passing gas means that your digestive tract is in working condition... And, I must admit, at times, gas is pretty darn funny!

O-kay, so it's out in the open: I'm a boy, too.

But what can you do? It's pointless to fight them. I've tried implementing a gag order on flatulence (insert your own tasteless joke here), but had no way of enforcing it. Passing gas is a very normal human body function, and gives us guys a common bond. We're farters.

Bunking with fifteen or so adolescent boys, it's a given. Someone is going to have gas. If you're not fortunate enough to be the one, you may as well put on your military issue gas mask and prepare for the worst. Or, you can always head to the kitchen and prepare your own counter-attack. It's biological warfare at its finest.

Everyone knows that if one "toot" elicits a snicker, two should be a hoot. And three? Three could incite a riot!

Some might think that this isn't fair to someone with, let's say, gastrointestinal control. Maybe so, but it's every boy for himself. If you chose to pass by the burrito bar without loading up, it's your own fault, and you will be penalized.

I've heard that if your nose is exposed to a foul odor for long enough it will shut down its receptors and you won't notice the odor anymore. I'm here to tell you that is bunk, a scientific hoax. I urge any scientist to spend the night sealed in a cabin with fifteen boys on taco night! Their opinion might sway. They can do a double-blind study, or whatever research they deem necessary, and, when the results are tabulated, I'm sure they'll agree: Boys are disgusting!

And, of course, farts are funny.

Warning: *(which should have been at the beginning of the chapter...whoops!)*

This chapter is not for everyone. The material herein involves boys doing "boy things." Not to say that girls aren't qualified, they just seem to have higher standards of decency. (Most of the time, anyway.) If you are not, or have never been, a boy, you may be offended and wish to skip over this chapter entirely. Read at your own discretion.

Thank you.

Bob's Mom-

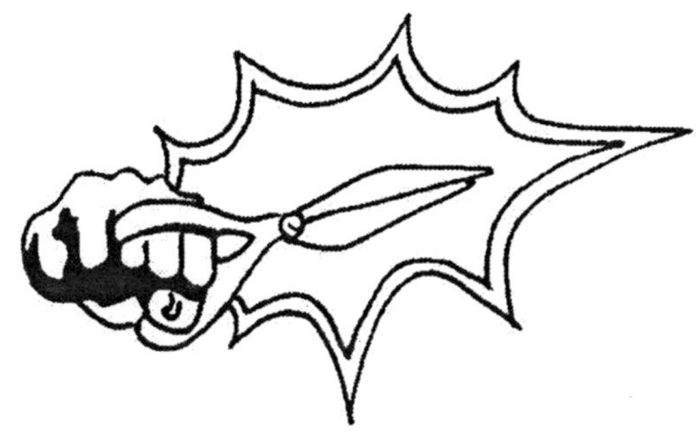

Real vs. Pretend

Sitting in the lodge, a lively conversation is developing over the lunch table. It centers around superheroes.

Specifically: If Superman and the Hulk team up and battle the entire group of X-Men—who will win?

Quite a weighty topic.

They go on to complicate things further: If Spiderman & Daredevil drop in—who'd win now?

"Bam!" "Pow!" "Kuh-bloom!"

The pros and cons are expertly debated at length.

Finally, an unassuming female camper chirps in from the far end of the table. "What if Zena the Warrior Princess was there?" A wide smile of satisfaction crosses her lips as a hush envelops the table.

The boy's minds are clearly at work.

But, after an apprehensive pause, her comment is dismissed, as one boy explains, "No, we're just talking about pretend superheroes."

At times, the lines dividing real and pretend can be blurry. I must admit, I often prefer the latter.

Superheroes? Snipe? Miracles?

Just what *is* real these days?

Superheroes have been discussed ad nausea. (See chapter one, four, six, and eleven, my pillowcase, my jammies, and the poster on my bedroom door...)

Although allusive little buggers, snipe have been spotted around camp, and I actually know a guy who received a nasty scratch from one. I've seen it!

Now miracles, there's something to chat about.

To define just what a miracle is, let's go back to our friendly eight-pound dictionary. (I promise I won't go into a rant this time.) Here goes—

Miracle: A marvelous event occurring within human experience, which cannot have been brought about by human power or by the operation of any natural agency, and must, therefore, be ascribed to the special intervention of a Deity or of some supernatural being; chiefly, an act (e.g. of healing) exhibiting control over the laws of nature, and serving as evidence that the agent is either divine of specially favoured by God.

Some people tend to classify miracles strictly within a religious context. Others find miracles to be supernatural, or some combination of both. Either way, most believe miracles to be about as uncommon as they come.

Not to step on any toes, but I think miracles are common. Quite common, actually. I believe miracles happen all around us each and every day. Some of them, anyway.

Let's look at a few things we sometimes take for granted: The sun came up this morning, as it did yesterday, and likely will tomorrow. We can say we understand how this happens, but can we make it happen? I don't think so. It's miraculous.

With all the viruses, bacteria, and diseases around, it's astounding that we don't get sick more frequently than we do. In most cases our immune systems take care of us. It's a complex system of actions and reactions that even doctors can't totally explain. It's an on-going miracle.

Ryan wasn't quite three when a baseball-sized tumor was discovered behind his left eye. His parents were told that he wouldn't likely survive the complicated surgery, which was expected to last twelve hours. Ryan's parents prayed. When the doctors went in to surgically remove it, they found nothing. No tumor. Without medical intervention, the tumor had shrunk—smaller, smaller, smaller—until "poof" it was gone. The doctors could give no medical rational for its disappearance. It was a miracle.

Take breathing. You breathe in, you breathe out. Most of the time you don't think about it—you just do it. The air enters your lungs and oxygen is removed and mixed into your bloodstream. The oxygen rich blood travels throughout your body nourishing various organs, including your brain. Yet, you rarely think *breathe in, breathe out; breathe in, breathe out*, and you never put any thought into all those other things happening. They just do. And it's truly a miracle it all works out.

Speaking of brains, we're told we only use about ten percent of ours. Only ten percent! So what's going on in the other ninety percent of mine? I don't know. Scientists don't know. In fact, scientists don't really understand how so many ridiculously complicated functions can possibly originate from that little pink slab of meat between your ears. (No, I'm not referring to Spam!)

And a single human cell contains so much information within its DNA that it would fill one thousand volumes with six hundred pages each. That's six-hundred-thousand pages of information from just one cell. Miraculous!

Not to mention all those crazy endocrine glands, and organs, and enzymes, and chemical reactions, and—

Even with all the progress we've made, there are so many things that science just can't explain.

Miracles.

According to the laws of aerodynamics, it's been scientifically proven that bumblebees are incapable of flight. Seriously! The ratio of their body's weight to their wingspan is so disproportionate that, according to science, bumblebees can't fly!

The conundrum was presented in scientific journals over seventy years ago, and, since then, scientists, engineers, and high school teachers have spent many hours studying and hypothesizing on the subject. Fortunately, bumblebees don't go to school, or read science journals. They just keep buzzing around, going about their own business.

Bottom line, medical science does not presently hold all the answers for us.

Not long ago, many in the U.S. pooh-poohed anything not of the Western "scientific" approach to healthcare. Today, practices such as visualization have proven to be an effective tool and are commonly taught to patients. One common approach used with children is to imagine a little Pac-Man eating away at their cancer. Multiple variations of visualizing the cancer shrinking or dissolving have been used with good results. After a treatment, some patients use a technique of relaxing in a warm tub and imagining their cancer cells swirling down the drain with the old water.

A mix of new approaches to health, and ancient practices from around the globe, have found their way into mainstream America. Teaming up with Western medical technology, these alternative therapies have become increasingly popular in fighting disease.

Herbal therapies, Traditional Chinese Medicine, energy medicine, antioxidants, biofeedback, acupuncture, meditation, Ayurvedic medicine, vitamins, detoxifications, Qi Gong, vibrational healing practices, immunological therapies, guided imagery, and harmonic devices are just of few of the approaches labeled holistic. Many boast of impressive results.

We are due for another monumental leap in medicine. Although none have delivered a sure-fire cure as of yet, new treatments and approaches are being developed, and new breakthroughs are certain. When we do find the cure, be it allopathic or holistic, there's no doubt it will also require a leap of faith.

It's just a matter of time.

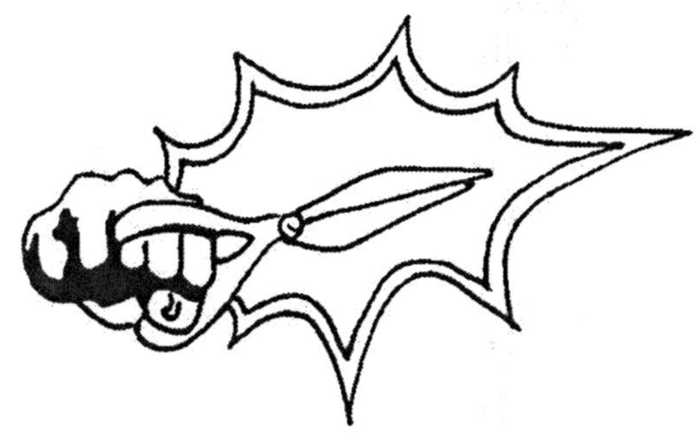

...& Not Another Word About Spam

Although these are just a smattering of the tens-of-thousands of children who have won the battle against childhood cancer, I believe these incredible kids are a fair sampling. Camp Sunrise is a truly magical place, but, quite possibly, no more than the various other oncology camps across the country. Likewise, Camp Sunrise boasts of true superheroes and genuinely miraculous children, but no more than other camps, hospitals, and organizations working with childhood cancer survivors.

These children, like all of us, will be adults one day. They will be in charge of directing our future. I hope you, like me, find great comfort in this. If there's one thing these distinguished sages and superheroes can teach us, it's that life is made not of problems, but of dreams. And who better to show us that those dreams are obtainable?

The children of Arizona Camp Sunrise have so much to teach, and the rest of us have so much to learn. If we can glean anything from their lives and stories, I hope it is that we mustn't squander and waste our moments, and to more fully appreciate life—every, every day.

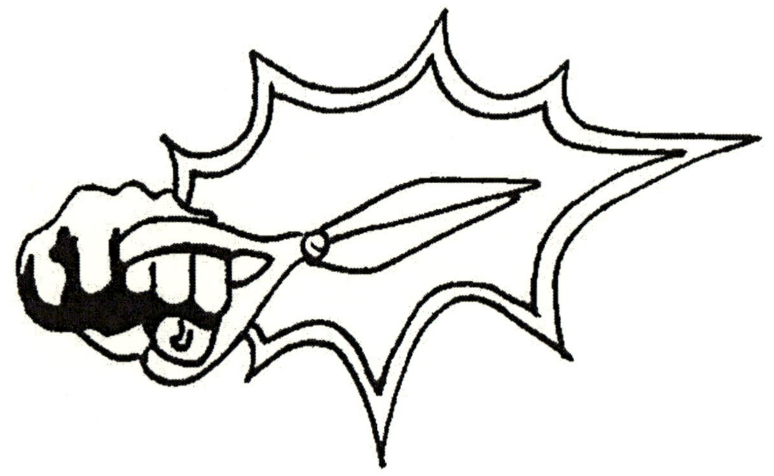

Credits/Contacts

To order additional copies of this book go to:
www.flyingwithscissors.com
or call: 1-800-865-1582

For information on donating to Arizona Camp Sunrise
call: 1-800-865-1582, or go to:
www.flyingwithscissors.com

"I Spoke as a Child" – Todd Daniel Snider
Lyrics used by permission:
Bro 'N Sis Music, Inc.
& Keith Sykes Music
Available on: *Todd Snider/Songs for the Daily Planet*

"Woman With the Strength of 10,000 Men" –
Peter Himmelman
Lyrics used by permission of artist
1991 Geffen Music/Himmasongs (ASCAP)
Available on: *Peter Himmelman/*
From Strength to Strength

Cover art by Randall J. Johnsen (aka Arjay)
Contact: goombert@aol.com

Formatting and computer technology by Jason
Poulter
Contact: polt@snaptek.com

Author contact:
www.flyingwithscissors.com
or: Bob Wallace
PO Box 2209
Sedona, AZ 86339-2209
bobwallace@flyingwithscissors.com

Printed in the United States
40382LVS00007B/235-1209